Robert Radin

NOCHE TRISTE

A Memoir of Anorexia

Edition Noëma

Bibliographic information published by the Deutsche Nationalbibliothek
Die Deutsche Nationalbibliothek lists this publication in the Deutsche Nationalbibliografie; detailed bibliographic data are available in the Internet at http://dnb.d-nb.de.

Bibliografische Information der Deutschen Nationalbibliothek
Die Deutsche Nationalbibliothek verzeichnet diese Publikation in der Deutschen Nationalbibliografie; detaillierte bibliografische Daten sind im Internet über http://dnb.d-nb.de abrufbar.

ISBN-13: 978-3-8382-0903-6
© *ibidem*-Verlag, Stuttgart 2023

For Amy and Max

Table of Contents

Part One:
The Nutrition Almanac

1. June 1978

It was cruise night on Van Nuys Boulevard and my friend Neil Baumgarten was heading over in his Nova SS and wanted me to ride shotgun.

I didn't like cruise night. The glare of the streetlights. The Fords and Chevys with their chrome blower stacks. The bikers standing outside Arby's, their choppers lined up at the curb. The girls driving in and out of the Bob's Big Boy parking lot with their feathered blonde hair and their blue eyeshadow and their lip gloss and their tube tops and their zip-around jeans. But Neil was my best friend back then, so I said I would go.

I showed up at his house a few minutes early and his father invited me in. He told me Neil was still getting ready and I should wait in the foyer.

I saw Neil's sister sitting on the couch in the living room. The curtains were drawn. Her mother was talking to her quietly, but it seemed like she wasn't listening.

I realized I had walked in on a family scene I wasn't supposed to be seeing. Part of me wanted to leave but part of me wanted to stay so I could make eye contact with Neil's sister, so I could exchange a look that would tell her how I felt, let her know I was in love with her and that whatever it was she was going through I would be there for her. But she just stared off into the dark of the room.

Neil finally came out of the bathroom and we went outside and stood on his lawn and looked up at the sky. The clouds were mackerel, that deep-red shimmer everyone attributed to the high concentrations of carbon monoxide and soot in the air.

Sorry about that, Neil said. My sister has this disease. It's called anorexia nervosa.

For many years these words would remain as strange and beautiful to me as they were that night, sounding more like the Latin name for a flower than a once-rare illness.

She can't eat, he said. She keeps losing weight.

I asked him questions but he couldn't give me answers. I imagined anorexia as some sort of virus that was eating his sister's flesh from the inside, but it wasn't a virus; it wasn't something you could catch. Yet she was dissolving. She was wasting away.

We got in the car and drove over to Van Nuys Boulevard. When we were at the light at Kittridge a couple of girls pulled up next to us in a black Trans Am. They looked a little older than us, like maybe they'd already graduated from high school. The driver was checking Neil out. He rolled down his window.

I'm a male gynecologist, he said.

This was his standard pick-up line. He thought it was a double entendre.

The driver leaned over her friend. She had a messy henna-colored mane and sharp teeth. She looked like a vampire.

I'm Mona, she said. This is Gretchen. You guys want to go park somewhere?

We followed them across Ventura Boulevard, into the hills, and stopped on a dead-end street. Neil pulled up the emergency brake.

They're into us, he said. So none of your bullshit.

He was referring to my habit of bringing up unsexy subjects at sexy times.

Fine, I said.

We got out of the car. Neil walked over to the Trans Am and talked to Mona for a few minutes. Then Gretchen got out and he slid into her seat and closed the door.

Gretchen approached me with a look of resignation. She had the same tangle of hair that Mona had, but she wasn't a vampire.

Let's get in your car, she said.

But it's nice out, I said.

We sat down on the sidewalk under a streetlamp.

I've been thinking about anorexia nervosa, I said. Have you heard of it?

It's when a girl starves herself, Gretchen said.

I was confused. Neil hadn't described it like that.

I know someone who has it, I said.

Gretchen drew her knees to her chest.

Mona's going to fuck your friend, she said. So we might as well do something.

As we drove home that night Neil told me he got to third base with Mona.

She knows what she's doing, he said. I'm definitely going to see her again. Do you want to make it a double?

No, I said.

So you're going to stay a virgin the rest of your life?

That's the plan.

We drove past the Busch brewery. The red light on the south building was flashing, which meant they were boiling the malt. I rolled down the window and breathed in the hops. It was my favorite smell in the world.

I wonder if your sister's still up, I said.

Stop talking about my sister, he said.

2. September 1978

I met Julia in Miss Ushijima's 2-D art class. She sat by herself in the front of the room and I sat in the back with a group of stoners. I didn't smoke pot but I knew if I sat with them Miss Ushijima would expect less of me.

Miss Ushijima was an odd bird. She was a gardener as well as a painter and would show up to class with dirt clods in her hair. She taught us color theory and how to blend and cross-hatch and stipple. I did a watercolor of a deer and a charcoal drawing of a potted plant. Miss Ushijima stood next to me and watched what I was doing, smelling of soil and dill, never saying a word.

Julia wore jeans and baggy sweatshirts, but I could see the tendons in her neck and the hollows at her jawbone. I would stare at her for half the class but she never looked up from what she was doing. Every once in a while she would go up to Miss Ushijima and ask a question in a barely audible voice; then she would walk back to her table, her head down and her shoulders hunched.

Miss Ushijima held a workshop at the end of each week. A couple of students would share their work in progress and ask the class for feedback. The week it was my turn I drew a tennis ball from three perspectives. My classmates mistook it for a baseball.

For her workshop Julia showed us a pencil drawing of a mother giving her young daughter a bath. Both the mother and the daughter were looking down into the tub, so you couldn't see their eyes. This gave the drawing a certain intimacy. I still remember the detail in the mother's housedress, the large cuffs at the sleeve, the buttons up the front. And I remember the mother's hair, the way Julia was able to show the weight of it, pulled back in a bun, and the daughter's hair, shining wet and plastered to her cheek.

It was inspired by Mary Cassatt, Julia said.

The class mumbled something. Nobody knew who Mary Cassatt was.

One morning we were drawing landscapes with pastels and I decided I needed olive green. I could have asked the stoners, but there was a good chance they had eaten theirs. Instead I pretended I needed to sharpen a pencil, and on my way back to my seat I made a detour to Julia.

I'm wondering if you have an olive green I might borrow, I said.

Julia searched my face to make sure I was trustworthy. Then she reached under the table and pulled out a small wooden case. She opened it and inside were trays of pastels, arranged by color and shade. They were so perfect, lined up next to each other like that, still in their paper wrappers. I felt the way I had as a kid when I opened up a new box of crayons. I didn't want to use them; I just wanted to look at them.

Julia picked out the olive green while I studied the landscape she was working on. The trees were blue and the mountains were red and the sky was a swirl of orange and yellow.

It's inspired by Art Nouveau, she said.
I love his work, I said.

When Julia stopped coming to class I searched for her in the hallways during passing periods and on the quad during lunch, but she was nowhere to be seen. I asked Miss Ushijima what had happened to her but she wouldn't — or couldn't — tell me anything.

3. January 1979

I decided I should bulk up. I'd always been skinny and felt self-conscious about it. No one kicked sand in my face, but a football player had kicked in the door to my locker.

I started going to the weight room during gym class. I'd never lifted weights before, so for the first few weeks I just watched other guys run through their circuits on the Universal machines and copied what they did. But after a couple of months they were all more massive than before and I looked pretty much the same. I couldn't understand it. It was like we were different species.

Then I met Clay. He appeared out of nowhere one morning, standing in front of the full-length mirror in nothing but a pair of white tennis shorts, doing tricep curls, staring at his reflection. He looked like a centurion: His hair was brown and shiny and perfectly feathered and he had a Roman nose and a jutting jaw. I could tell that he'd been skinny once too, but somehow he'd defined his body. There was a deep cleft in his chest and his arms and legs were cut with muscle. As he pulled up the barbell he exhaled in short, determined bursts. His face turned red. He looked like he was going to cry.

The whole thing was unnerving. I'd never been able to look at myself in the mirror like that, with that much pride and that much purpose. I went over to the leg-extension machine and began my workout. I lifted the weight level with my hip and lowered it back down. Within a few minutes Clay was standing next to me, waiting for his turn. I felt like I had to work harder with him standing there, to show him I had as much right to the machine as he did.

You should do more weight, he said.

He knelt down behind the bench and adjusted the weight pin.

Try that, he said.

I could immediately feel the strain in my quads.

Do ten of those, he said. Then rest a minute and do ten more.

I thought my quads were going to seize on me, but when I was finished it felt like my legs had doubled in size.

Clay set the pin at 200 and lay down on the bench.

Oh shit, I thought. He's going to do the leg curl. I contemplated running away.

The leg curl was the one exercise I'd never seen anyone do, because to do it you had to lie face down on the bench, brace the back of your heels against the pulley arm, and lift the weight with your hamstrings, and to do that you had to rotate your pelvis in a way that made it look like you were fucking the bench. But Clay didn't care.

We started working out together. Clay had his regimen and I followed along. On Mondays, Wednesdays, and Fridays we did bench press, biceps curls, triceps curls, wrist curls, flies, lat-pulls, military press, shoulder press, skullcrushers, chin-ups, and dips. On Tuesdays and Thursdays we did leg press, hamstring press, squats, calf raises, deltoid raises, toe raises, inner-thigh lifts, knee extensions, and sit-ups. We worked out with free weights as much as possible because Clay said they gave you more definition and were a better measurement of real strength.

He explained to me the way muscle mass was built: The muscle tissue tore when you lifted something heavy. When it mended its mass was increased and strengthened. That was why you weren't supposed to work the same muscle group every day, because the muscles needed time to heal. Working out was this gradual process of breaking the muscle down and building it back up. The burning you felt was from the lactic acid. You wanted that burn — when you felt it you knew you were building muscle.

Feel the burn, Clay would say. And though I didn't really believe what he was telling me, though I thought it was a crude explanation for something that had to be much more complicated, I did what he said and made my body burn as he stood over me and yelled at me: *Come on, one more rep, come on motherfucker, come on, one more, one more, one more.*

My shirts were getting tighter. Sometimes I'd dare to look at myself in the mirror before I left the locker room, and I could see it was happening: I was developing Clay's body.

The day Clay first bench-pressed 300 pounds he invited me to his house that night to watch *Dog Day Afternoon*.

It's never been on television before, he said.

When I got to his house he introduced me to his parents. His mother was sitting on the couch, crocheting an afghan. His father was in the kitchen, hunched over the dining table, fiddling with a circuit board. He shook my hand and showed me a drawing he'd made on a paper napkin. It looked like a man screaming into his own ear, but he explained it was a diagram for a device he was making that would stop kids from siphoning gas from his car at night. He'd hook a motion detector to the gas cap, then run a circuit to the horn, the windshield wipers, and the headlights, and put everything on a timer, so it would all go off at once.

You could just park the car in the garage, Clay said.

I'm not changing my life around for a bunch of hoodlums, his father said.

Clay and I went to his bedroom. Like the rest of the house, it was done up in Country American, with yellow wainscoting and blue gingham wallpaper. There was a desk, a bed, and a little television on the night table. The only real sign of Clay's presence was the poster of *Pumping Iron* taped to his closet door.

He'd made a big bowl of popcorn and grabbed a six-pack of 7-Up. We sat on the bed and turned on the TV. He asked me if I loved Pacino and I said I did, even though I'd never seen a Pacino movie before. Not even *The Godfather*.

The soda made us gassy. We belched when Sonny's mother was begging him to turn himself in, and again when Sonny was checking the limousine for weapons. When Sal died I started crying. Clay didn't say anything.

When the movie was over Clay turned off the TV and went to his desk and opened the top drawer and took out a red envelope.

I got you this card, he said.

He handed me the envelope. The flap was sealed so tight I had to tear it from the corner.

The outside of the card had a picture of two men on horseback. They were wearing black breeches and red doublets and floppy hats. One of the men was pointing at something in the distance. I remember thinking they were from Renaissance times, which for me covered everything between the Middle Ages and the Industrial Revolution. The card was blank on the inside. I didn't know why he was giving it to me, but I thanked him.

I knew you would like it, he said.

The next day there was a girl with purple hair in the weight room. She was on crutches, her right leg in a cast up to her thigh. She sat down on the bench press and the football coach introduced her.

Listen up, he said. This is Elsa. She broke her leg, so she's going to be with us for a while.

Everyone held back their snickering until the coach had left. The color of Elsa's hair meant she was a punk, and punks were lepers. I approached her and offered to show her how to use the upper-body machines. She thanked me but told me she was just there to kill time. Then she took a copy of *Valley of the Dolls* out of her backpack and started to read.

A few days later Elsa had a friend with her, a girl with spiky hair and lots of eyeliner. They were sitting on the bench press, talking about Bowie. Elsa said her mother had been obsessed with him but lost all interest after he abandoned his Ziggy persona. When Clay and I asked them if they wouldn't mind moving Elsa introduced me to her friend.

This is Nicole, she said.

Nicole and I shook hands.

He said he would teach me how to lift weights, Elsa said.

The two girls started laughing.

The offer still stands, I said.

I love your hair, Nicole said.

She likes skinny boys, Elsa said.

So do you, Nicole said.

We need to get going here, Clay said.

They moved to the leg-press machine and Clay and I began our set. But the whole time he was yelling at me to do one more rep, just one more, just one more, I was thinking about Nicole. I hoped she'd return to the weight room at some point so I could get to know her better, but it never happened.

When I got to the weight room the next day Clay had started without me. I asked him what was going on. He told me he didn't want to work out together anymore.

I don't think you're serious, he said.

But we're lifting five times a week, I said.

I don't know why you're doing this in the first place.

I didn't have a good answer for him. The truth was I didn't know. I started lifting weights because I thought that's what men did, to make themselves look like men, to make themselves attractive to women. I'd never enjoyed it, but I kept doing it because I looked up to Clay and wanted to stay friends with him.

Get out of my face, he said.

I was devastated. We kept our distance from each other after that, timing our workouts so we were never in the same part of the weight room at the same time. But my interest was flagging. I stayed with it for a while to prove to Clay that he was wrong, but I just couldn't push myself without him. I lifted less weight, did fewer reps, until my body went back to the way it was before. And then I stopped going to the weight room altogether.

4. September 1981

I dropped out of college after my freshman year and took the first job I could get, winding stator coils for three-phase induction motors for elevator hoists. On the weekends I delivered flowers for a nursery called the Plant Peddler.

My first delivery was a bouquet of pink roses for a woman named Fiona Stewart. She was the manager of an old movie theater on Ventura Boulevard. As I walked into the lobby I was filled with nostalgia: This was where I'd first seen *Willy Wonka & the Chocolate Factory*.

I saw Nicole at the concession counter. She was wearing a blue pantsuit and a matching bowtie. As I approached her I could see she didn't remember me, but she was beaming at the sight of the bouquet, so I gave it to her. Then she opened the card.

This isn't for me, she said.

She gave the bouquet back to me and went to get Fiona Stewart, who returned visibly pissed.

You need to check before you give someone flowers, she said.

I felt terrible. I wasn't sure if I was only going to make matters worse, but I drove back to the Plant Peddler and wrapped a dozen Gerbera daisies in green tissue paper and returned to the theater and gave them to Nicole.

On our first date Nicole and I went to the Norton Simon Museum. As we stood looking at Degas' *The Laundress* she told me it reminded her of something her best friend would paint.

Her name is Julia, she said. She has anorexia. Do you know what that is?

I couldn't believe they knew each other. It took me a moment to respond.

I think so, I said.

She's in the hospital, she said. It's her third time.

I didn't tell Nicole that I knew Julia. I felt like admitting this was as good as admitting I'd liked Julia, or, I feared, still liked her. I didn't want my feelings for Julia to interfere with my feelings for Nicole, even as I held out hope that, through Nicole, I might get to see Julia again.

5. October 1981

Nicole and I took a day trip to Tijuana. We walked up and down the Avenida Revolución with the other tourists, stopping into the various souvenir shops to watch people shake maracas, play with marionettes, and haggle over serapes. We got lunch from a taco cart. We drank Mexican beer.

It was a festive scene, but it changed that night, when all the families disappeared and were replaced by teenage girls who'd come down to Tijuana to get drunk for the first time. They staggered around the Avenida, the low riders calling to them from their cars. But it was the American men they needed to worry about: They were standing outside the nightclubs, smoking cigarettes, waiting.

Nicole found the whole scene distressing and wanted to leave, so we took a cab to the border. We got through customs fast, but had to wait an hour for the trolley back to National City, where we'd parked our car.

Not long after we got on the train I broke into a sweat and started experiencing painful stomach cramps. We got off at the Chula Vista station and I ran to the bathroom, but it was locked for the night.

I knew I was going to shit myself and didn't want Nicole — or anyone else — to see me, so I crossed the train tracks and climbed the guardrail and ran as far and as fast as I could, away from the lights and the cars, until I was lost in an empty lot, one of the long stretches of chaparral between the train tracks and the freeway.

I was too sick to make the drive back to Los Angeles, so we checked into a motel in National City and I lay in bed for the next two days, getting up every five minutes to go to the bathroom. Nicole kept me hydrated and entertained, bringing me glasses of water or cans of juice, reading me articles from her fashion magazines. I remember a piece about how you could find renewed potential in your closet cast-offs. The trick, the writer said, was to repurpose your dresses as skirts and your blouses as shirts. And I remember a photo of an anorexic model who was wearing a blue scoop-neck sweater. The shadows at her collarbone were deep, shocking.

On the third day my symptoms began to abate, and I felt a bit more energy. Nicole brought me an English muffin from the breakfast buffet, and a bowl of Cheerios and a banana, but when I asked her if I could have a cinnamon roll she said no, because she thought it might upset my stomach.

That evening we went to the pool and waded around in the shallow end for a bit; then Nicole asked if she could pick me up.

Please, she said.

She cradled me in her arms and carried me to the deep end, pretending the water had given her super strength, until her feet could no longer touch the bottom and she was laughing so hard that she had to let me go.

When we got back to Los Angeles I stayed at her apartment for a few days, just so she could continue to nurse me. She gave me bowls of white rice and glasses of ginger ale.

She had a scale in her bathroom, between the toilet and the sink, and one night after we'd finished brushing our teeth I pulled it out and stepped on it.

I've lost 10 pounds, I said.

She looked at me in the mirror.

You're so handsome, she said.

When I was growing up I used to ask my mother if I was ugly. *You're not ugly, but you're certainly not handsome*, she'd say, and I thought her equivocation was exactly right.

There was something wrong with my face. Each of my features was fine in isolation, but not taken together. The whole was less than the sum of its parts. I'd been standing in front of bathroom mirrors my entire life, hoping to change that, hoping that, through the act of staring at myself, I could will myself into the person I wanted to be, make my nose smaller, my mouth more defined, my jaw more angular, until my profile was perfect.

That night, standing on the scale in Nicole's bathroom, I saw, for a moment, what she saw, my reflection through her eyes. But then the moment passed, and I wanted to get it back, and I thought I could, if I just lost a little more weight. I could make my eyes a little bit bigger, the planes of my face a little bit sharper.

Steven Levenkron, the therapist who treated Karen Carpenter, published his young-adult novel, *The Best Little Girl in the World*, in 1978. ABC made it into a television movie in 1981, casting a young Jennifer Jason Leigh in the lead role. They would rebroadcast the movie many times in the months after Karen Carpenter died.

I didn't see it, but I remember the commercial for it: Leigh, painfully thin, stares at herself in the mirror and sees an overweight person reflected back at her.

For years this was the defining image of anorexia. It represented, in purely visual terms, how an anorexic person felt. But it was itself a distortion, because while it captured something true about anorexia — the deep sense of shame, the self-hatred — it simultaneously simplified it so that people wouldn't have to acknowledge the more disturbing complexities of the illness. Because the truth of the mirror — that habitual, compulsive staring at yourself — isn't that you see yourself as fat, but that you see yourself as beautiful, or handsome, or whatever it is you wish you were, and there's no visual shorthand for this, no sympathetic way to portray it at all.

6. November 1981

Sometimes I think it began two weeks later, when I was feeling better and Nicole and I went to Angela's Ristorante. It was our favorite pizza place. It had red leather booths and lattice archways strung with plastic grapes, and a mural on the wall that depicted the journey of the grape from the vine to the bottle, complete with images of people stomping out purple juice in a big wooden tub and oak barrels stacked on racks in a dark cellar.

A young man greeted us as we sat down. He told us his name was Bruce and that he would be our busboy for the evening. His curly hair was cut in the shape of a hedge.

If you need anything please don't hesitate, he said.

Nicole was wearing a snug V-neck sweater and Bruce was looking at her chest.

That will be all, Bruce, I said.

Bruce returned to the kitchen.

I washed dishes at an Italian restaurant and I never introduced myself to the customers, I said.

That's different, Nicole said. The dishwasher is behind the scenes.

The busboy and the dishwasher are a team, I said.

The waitress gives the busboy a percentage of her tips, she said.

But she always shortchanges him, I said. And he becomes bitter, and he turns to the dishwasher for comfort.

When our waitress came we ordered the same thing we always ordered: a small antipasto and a large mushroom pie. I ate the antipasto without giving it a second thought, scarfing down slices of salami and spearing garbanzo beans with my fork. But when the pizza came something changed: I imagined the cheese congealing inside me, sitting in my intestines, toxic, rotting.

I'm not hungry, I said.

Nicole and I had an unspoken agreement: When we went out for pizza we synchronized our eating, to make sure we got an equal number of pieces and neither of us felt like more of a glutton than the other. So if I didn't have any pizza, then neither could she.

Just have one slice, she said.

Fine, I said.

She broke off a slice and put it on my plate. I waited for it to cool and took a bite, chewing and chewing and chewing, hoping that maybe if I masticated the cheese into a pulp it wouldn't be as fattening.

Bruce the busboy walked past us. He was delivering three glasses of water on a silver tray to the family in the next booth, a father and his two daughters.

One of the daughters looked like she was in grade school. The other was a teenager with an ample bosom. Just as Bruce reached their table his left leg buckled and the tray tilted and the glasses slid off, the water arcing through the air and falling in sheets on the teenage girl's chest.

Bruce righted himself.

I'm so sorry, he said.

The father looked like he was going to swallow his tongue. The younger girl laughed.

It's okay, the teenage girl said.

Bruce ran back to the kitchen and returned with a stack of towels and a red chef's jacket. He gave the jacket to the teenage girl.

You can change in the bathroom, he said. And I want you all to know you're eating free tonight, so please order whatever you want. I highly recommend the manicotti.

Nicole leaned toward me.

He did it on purpose, she said.

But I couldn't pay attention to Bruce just then, because I knew I was never coming back to Angela's, because I knew I was never eating pizza again.

7. December 1981

When Julia got out of the hospital her friend Kate had a small get-together at her parents' house to welcome her home. Kate's family lived in the hills above Chatsworth, in a chalet at the end of a dirt road.

Kate greeted me and Nicole at the door when we arrived and led us into the living room. Her parents were there, sitting on the sofa, sipping wine. Julia was with them. She wore a long green dress and a heavy blue cardigan. She looked even thinner than she had in high school.

I introduced myself to everyone. Julia showed no sign of remembering me. It was disconcerting to think how forgettable I was.

I sat on the sofa next to Nicole and took in the room: It had a cathedral ceiling, and a stone fireplace, and a huge built-in entertainment center, and a wall of windows facing north, looking out at the Santa Susana Mountains.

Your house is so beautiful, I said.

We like it, Kate's father said.

There was a tall, cylindrical object next to the entertainment center. It was covered with a dark baffle.

That's a nice speaker, I said.

It's not a speaker, Kate's father said. It's an ionizer.

He considered me for a moment and decided I had no idea what he was talking about.

It creates negative ions, he said, which in turn remove particulates from the air. Because there are two layers to an atom: the nucleus, which consists of protons and neutrons packed tightly together, and the more fluid outer layer, consisting of electrons. There always has to be an equal number of protons to electrons, a balance between the inside and the outside. An ion is just an electrically charged atom. You create an ion by either adding electrons or taking them away. If you add electrons, the ion is positive; if you take them away, it's negative. This machine sends out an electromagnetic pulse that creates negative ions, and these negative ions then collide with airborne particles like dust, pollen, bacteria, smoke — you name it — creating a new, negatively charged particle, and this negatively charged particle keeps attracting positive particles until it becomes so heavy that it drops out of the air.

I thought of all those evenings when I was growing up, sitting on the couch after I'd made dinner, waiting for my mother to get home from work, watching the light from the setting sun fill our living room, revealing all the dust motes floating around me, and how I just sat there, breathing them in. I wondered now if the damage was irreparable.

We hear you got sick in Tijuana, Kate's mother said.

I think I had dysentery, I said.

Ah yes, Kate's father said. Montezuma's revenge.

But we both had chicken tacos, Nicole said.

Heat usually kills the E. coli, Kate's father said.

I wondered whether my chicken had been sitting around longer than Nicole's. Maybe the guy at the taco cart had piled the new chicken on top of the old chicken, thinking the new chicken would heat the old chicken, and kill whatever bacteria had come back, but it hadn't worked.

We moved out to the backyard for dinner. Kate's mother had set a beautiful table on the deck, overlooking her flower garden. Her azaleas were still in bloom.

I've prepared a Barcelonian meal, she said. Cold gazpacho with pan con tomate for starters, followed by tortillas española, paella with fresh shrimp and crayfish, and escudella, a hot soup with beef and beans and potatoes. We will eat in the Spanish style.

I didn't know what that meant. I waited to pick up my spoon.

I spent my junior year in Barcelona, she said. We took classes in the mornings and spent the afternoons at the cafés eating *tapas* and drinking wine with our professors. Then we'd all pile into a taxi and go to *La Sagrada Familia*. It turns out Gaudi was a devout Catholic. He didn't care if he ever finished the cathedral; the cathedrals that inspired him — Reims and Laon — were never finished either. He just kept working on it, his whole life, continually changing the style, each change corresponding to some form of personal upheaval. You can see it in the transept as it gets higher and higher. It's like you're reading a man's diary.

I felt so intimidated by Kate's parents. They were so cosmopolitan, so confident as they held forth on a range of subjects. I wondered how such people came to be.

Kate's mother poured everyone a glass of wine.

This is from a small winery south of Barcelona, she said. It's full-bodied and pairs well with the paella.

The only thing I knew about wine was that sometimes it was red and sometimes it was white.

I took a sip. It was so bitter I wanted to spit it out.

Julia picked at her plate, ate at the edges of things, paused forever between each bite.

This is delicious, she said. You must give me the recipe for the omelet.

It's really simple, Kate's mother said.

So it's an omelet after all, I said. You called it a tortilla. I thought I was missing something.

This isn't Mexican food, Kate's father said.

Right, I said.

He considered me again, and concluded, again, that I had no idea what he was talking about.

The dishes Americans order in Mexican restaurants aren't Mexican, he said. They're American versions of Mexican food. They make use of some traditionally Mexican ingredients, but they're not Mexican.

After dinner Kate's parents retired for the night and we returned to the living room. Kate put on the new Joan Armatrading album. Nicole got up and the two of them danced. Julia sat still on the sofa, her hands folded in her lap.

I had a class with you in high school, I said.

Miss Ushijima's 2-D art, she said. You never gave me back my olive-green pastel.

I didn't think she'd remember me, and had been bracing myself for that, but now, instead, I felt guilty.

I promise I'll get you a new one, I said.

I replaced it a long time ago, she said.

I'm so sorry.

I'm teasing you.

We watched Kate and Nicole sway back and forth through the first verse of "I'm Lucky," the two of them lip-syncing the refrain.

I can walk under ladders ... I can walk under ladders ...

I asked Julia if she wanted to dance and she demurred, saying she didn't know how. But when the drums kicked in I insisted.

Come on, I said.

We went to the middle of the room and I took her hand and led her through a series of slow turns. She was graceful, but her body offered no resistance. It made it impossible for me to keep the rhythm — there was nothing for me to push against.

I led her into a cuddle position, then spun her away, but when I brought her back my hand accidentally slipped under her sweater. I could feel the bones in her back, the depressions between her vertebrae, and I felt like I had violated her, and wanted to take my hand away, but I didn't want to make her feel more self-conscious, so I waited until the song was over.

Nicole talked about Julia the whole way back to her apartment.

Her hands are purple, she said. Her collarbone is sticking out. Her thighs are smaller than her calves.

She was so angry that Julia had been discharged, because she hadn't gained any weight, and now she was living with her parents again, and that was only going to make things worse.

As I was brushing my teeth she came into the bathroom, clutching her copy of Hilde Bruch's *The Golden Cage: The Enigma of Anorexia Nervosa*, and read me a long passage about a young woman named Yvonne, whose mother had monitored her eating, and they fought about it constantly. When Yvonne went away to college she thought things would get better. She thought that, left to her own devices, she'd be able to start eating normally again, and would recover on her own, but instead things got worse. Every time she gained a few pounds she panicked, and took laxatives and diuretics to lose the new weight, until she became so dehydrated that she collapsed and was taken to the hospital, where they fed her intravenously, pumping her with electrolytes and glucose until they could transition her back to solid food. When her doctor told her he wanted her to stay in the hospital until her weight was safely above 80 pounds she screamed at him, and said he wanted her to hate herself, and demanded to be discharged.

Talking to a therapist doesn't work unless you're at a certain weight, Nicole said. Bruch says it's between 90 and 100 pounds, depending on your build.

This wasn't the first time she'd read me a passage from *The Golden Cage*. She'd told me the illness heightened your sensory perceptions, made the color of flowers brighter, the shapes of leaves and clouds more defined. She'd said you could exercise for five or six hours a day, running, swimming, biking, and it was like you were superhuman. In the beginning there was a rush from the increase in the endorphins, and you had more energy than you did before, and you could fool yourself into thinking your starving was making you stronger.

I hated it when she read to me from *The Golden Cage*, not because I objected to anything in the book itself, but because I found the cover so disturbing: It was an illustration of an emaciated woman, her long red hair tied back in a ponytail, her head craned forward, accentuating the line of her jaw and the length of her neck. Her skin was pinched tight at her cheekbones, her lips pursed. Her eyes were two hollows. Her head was inside a cage.

The Golden Cage meant everything to Nicole. She'd read a review of it in one of her magazines, and when it came out in paperback she bought a copy. By the time we started dating she'd read it so many times she'd practically committed it to memory. It helped her understand what Julia was going through. It helped her feel closer to her. It provided her some sort of solace.

8. February 1982

I bought a book called the *Nutrition Almanac*. I'd learned about it from Irving Pitkin, a nutritionist who had a weekly radio show on KPFK, the local Pacifica station. He consulted the book regularly while he was on air, reading from it as if it were a sacred text.

Pitkin preached the importance of *high-value foods*, the term he used to refer to food that had a high ratio of nutrients to calories. Brewer's yeast was, for him, the quintessential high-value food because it contained 16 amino acids, 17 vitamins, and 14 minerals, and was a great source of RNA.

My favorite part of the *Nutrition Almanac* was an illustration of a cross section of a kernel of wheat, magnified one hundred times to reveal the endosperm and the germ and the bran. I studied it as if it were a photo of the beginning of the universe.

I especially liked the word *kernel*. It made me think there was a heart of the matter, a truth that all things had at their center.

If that was true, then the germ was the truth of the truth, the best part of the kernel. It constituted only 2% of it, but that 2% was 64% thiamin, 26% riboflavin, 21% pyridoxine, 8% protein, 7% pantothenic acid, and 3% niacin.

But for me the real, radical value of the *Nutrition Almanac* was the table in the appendix. It listed the nutritive contents of every possible food, and I consulted it constantly, looking for substitutions, foods that would provide more protein with less fat, fewer carbohydrates, fewer calories. I went over the numbers in my head, searching for the perfect combination. Once I found it I could stop, I told myself. Then I wouldn't have to think about food at all anymore. Then all my thoughts would be directed to other things.

I began by making small adjustments, keeping a lot of the foods I was already eating. For breakfast I had a bowl of oatmeal with cinnamon, raisins, and lowfat milk. For lunch I had cottage cheese and a banana. For dinner I had a chicken breast, carrots, and brown rice. I drank eight glasses of water a day and four cups of orange juice from concentrate.

Total calories: 1,884
Total protein: 130.92 grams
Total fat: 32.44 grams

9. March 1982

The *Nutrition Almanac* taught me about amino acids — both what they were, and how important they were.

There were eight essential amino acids — essential because the body couldn't produce them, so it was necessary to get them from food. If one amino acid was missing, or present in a low amount, the body could convert that much less to protein.

To put it another way, a protein was only as good as its lowest essential amino acid. So if a food contained 100 percent of a person's lysine requirement but only 20 percent of her methionine requirement, then the body could use only 20 percent of the protein in that food. That's why the *Nutrition Almanac* recommended eating complementary foods in a meal — if a food was low in one amino acid, you could combine it with another food high in that amino acid. But I didn't want to get into any of that. I wanted to keep things as simple as possible.

The cottage cheese and chicken were complete sources of all the essential amino acids, but my diet had too much fat and too much sodium, so I made some changes. For breakfast I had oatmeal with cinnamon and raisins and substituted nonfat milk for lowfat milk. For lunch I had a banana and substituted nonfat yogurt for cottage cheese. For dinner I had brown rice and substituted soybeans for chicken and spinach for carrots. I drank eight glasses of water a day and reduced my orange-juice consumption from four cups to three.

Total calories: 1,531
Total protein: 60.25 grams
Total fat: 15.55 grams

10. April 1982

Because of the ratio of essential amino acids in the soybeans, only 46% could be converted into protein, and this worried me. I also felt like the food I was eating was just sitting in my intestines, turning toxic, rotting. I wanted to evacuate it as soon as possible, to get it out of my body for good. I needed more fiber.

For breakfast I had nonfat milk, substituted wheat germ and miller's bran for the oatmeal, and eliminated the raisins. For lunch I had nonfat yogurt and substituted an apple for the banana. For dinner I substituted two hardboiled eggs for the soybeans, cauliflower for the spinach, and bulgur for the brown rice. I drank eight glasses of water a day and reduced my orange-juice consumption from three cups to two.

Total calories: 1,303
Total protein: 97.15 grams
Total fat: 32.53 grams

11. May 1982

Once again I had too much fat in my diet, and now too much cholesterol, and only 54% of the eggs could be converted into protein, so I had to make more changes. For breakfast I cooked bran and millet in boiled water. For lunch I had a green apple. For dinner I had a can of tuna fish with bulgur and a stalk of raw broccoli. I drank eight glasses of water a day and reduced my orange-juice consumption from two cups to one. I knew the juice had too much sugar, but I couldn't give it up: I imagined the citric acid burning through me, disinfecting me, stripping me down to bone.

Total calories: 1,229
Total protein: 112.2 grams
Total fat: 14.8 grams

The hardest part of the day was when I finished dinner, when I took the last bite of food and knew I had nothing more to look forward to until morning.

Sometimes I woke in the middle of the night from a hunger pain, and I lay there in bed, smoothing the hollow of my abdomen with the heel of my hand, trying to change the pain into something else. I told myself that each spasm was cutting into the fat in my body. Each spasm was cutting away a little more of me.

12. August 1982

Nicole and I had been going to a revival house in Santa Monica two or three times a week, almost since we started dating. But I couldn't get through a film now without falling asleep. I'd feel fine when we got to the theater, but as soon as the lights went down I struggled to stay awake. I'd curse myself, and sit up straight, and grip the armrests of my seat, all to no avail. After a few minutes I'd relent and yield to the fatigue, making a show of slumping down as if I were in fact settling in, as if I were simply trying to find a more comfortable position.

I always woke just before the closing credits, so some part of me must have known what was going on, must have been aware of my surroundings, somehow attending, unconsciously, to the soundtrack, the voices, the music. I'd sit up slowly, casually, and wait for the lights to come up, and as Nicole and I walked out of the theater I'd tell her how much I loved the film, and speak with great conviction and specificity about the part I'd seen, the lighting, the composition, the sets, hoping I could bluff my way out, make her believe I'd been awake the whole time.

It made no sense, because she always knew I was lying. She'd play along at first, agree with all my observations, then ask me a question, pretend there was something she didn't understand, a plot point she knew I'd slept through, and I'd fudge, and say something vague, like *I think that's part of the director's aesthetic*. But then she'd press me on it, until I was caught out, and confessed, and she laughed, and told me she didn't care, but I felt terrible, because I was sleeping through some of the greatest films in the history of cinema.

At work it was no laughing matter. Every morning I had a box of stator cores waiting for me on my workbench, with a connection diagram, usually an overhead perspective of a stator core with its winding pattern, each phase represented by a different color — red, green, or blue.

Sometimes they gave me a developed diagram instead, and this took a minute to interpret, because it required me to imagine myself standing inside the stator bore, turning along its axis and looking outwards at each slot, until I'd turned 360° and seen all 36 slots — or 48 slots if it was a 48-slot stator — and this wasn't something I wanted to visualize for too long, as it conjured a kind of punishing, postindustrial panopticon, and made me panic.

I used 35-gauge copper wire most of the time. Each coil had two layers; I had to start the first layer at the bottom of the stator, and the second layer at the top. I used a tool that looked like a crochet hook, pulling the wire through a slot, across the teeth, and over to the next slot indicated on the connection diagram. So for the first layer of the first phase I might thread the wire up the starting slot, over two slots and down, over seven slots and up, back two slots and down, over nine slots and up, over two slots and down, over nine slots and up, and back two slots and down. I'd leave the lead loose, shift counterclockwise 120°, and start the first layer of the second phase.

This all took some concentration and visual acuity, because while the connection diagram was less distressing than the developed one, it didn't have numbers for the individual slots — maybe because it would've made the illustration too busy — so I had to identify the slot I was supposed to thread by sight, and if I got it wrong there wouldn't be a magnetic field, and if there was no magnetic field, the induction motor wouldn't work.

And that's what happened. I'd get to work and start winding and within minutes I just wanted to go to sleep. As my vision blurred I'd guess at the slots — educated guesses, I told myself, based on previous windings I'd done for a particular vendor. But really I was waiting for a moment when no one was around, and I could lay my head on the workbench and take a nap.

Near the end of each day someone came in from quality control and pulled a random stator to test. They'd connect the leads according to the correct polarities and series and phases, and if your stator failed they'd pull all your work for the day and test it, and if another one failed they'd dock your pay and place you in *performance study*, as they called it, which meant they were watching you.

When three of my stators failed my boss, Frank Cox, called me into his office and asked me what was going on.

You've been here almost a year and never had a stator fail, he said.

I've been having vision problems, I said.

He was dubious.

You don't look good, he said.

I just need to go to the eye doctor, I said.

The other winders reviled Mr. Cox, as did his peers on the management team, but I had a good relationship with him. It was in part because I never made mistakes, but it was also because he'd served in Vietnam and wanted to talk about it, and I wanted to listen, because Vietnam had changed everything forever and I wanted to understand what had happened.

I'm supposed to fire you, he said.

Please give me one more chance, sir, I said.

I can't keep you on the floor. That's out of the question.

I panicked. This was my sole source of income — I'd quit my weekend job out of exhaustion.

There might be another option, he said.

I'll do anything, sir, I said.

We've been having problems with some of the vendors. Stators going missing, or arriving stripped to the core. The bottom line is it's impacting our bottom line, so we're thinking about doing the delivery ourselves.

I can do that, sir. I have delivery experience.

So you know the city pretty well.

The truth was I knew only the Valley, but I lied.

Like the back of my hand, sir, I said.

Good, he said. This way I can keep you on. It's going to look like favoritism, and some people will be pissed. But I can deal with it if you can.

13. September 1982

Nicole thought I had anorexia and wanted me to see Marvin Kashner, the doctor who was treating Julia. I refused, though I think some part of me felt relieved, or vindicated, like I finally had her full, undivided attention. But I felt resentful too, because she'd been happy when I first started losing weight, and now, all of a sudden, she'd decided I was sick.

I told her I'd make an appointment with Irving Pitkin since I'd been wanting to see him anyway. He did private consultations — he gave out his phone number on air — but when I called him to schedule an appointment he sounded suspicious, and spoke in a hushed voice, and asked me what kind of car I drove.

Let's keep this brief, he said.

He gave me directions to his home that were over a page long and told me I had to follow them precisely. It was a circuitous route that doubled back on itself constantly. Finally I reached a side street near the beach, and drove up and down it seven times, because he hadn't given me his address, telling me instead he would watch for me. I was just about to go home when he emerged from a shady bungalow and hailed me down.

You made it, he said.

He looked nothing like I'd imagined him. I'd pictured Jack LaLanne in looser pants, but he was Burl Ives on a bender.

My apologies for the complicated instructions, he said. But I had to be sure no one was tailing you. I've been doing a study on the impact the second San Onofre reactor is having on groundwater in the area and the feds have me under surveillance. They've tapped my phone. You probably heard the clicking sound when we spoke.

I told him I had, even though I hadn't.

Please come in, he said.

I parked my car and followed him inside. He led me into his study and sat me down opposite him at his desk.

I go through this room every day to check for bugs, he said. So rest assured, we can speak freely. Now tell me how I can help.

I've been losing weight, I said. I just want to make sure I'm eating right.

How tall are you?

Six feet.

How much do you weigh?

I told him 120. I was really 100.

You're small-boned, he said. So ideally you should be between 145 and 155. But being too thin isn't necessarily a bad thing. You know, we're programmed to eat a lot of things that are unhealthy for us. The food industry is engaged in a campaign of disinformation. When you go to the supermarket you're caught in the vortex. But the good news is we have a tool for foiling the plot. It's called the *Nutrition Almanac*.

I have a copy, I said.

Then you're going to be okay.

I felt my eyes welling with tears. I blinked hard to make them go away.

He asked me if I fasted.

Whether it's for health, or religion, or as a form of social protest, you shouldn't do it for more than forty days, he said.

I don't fast, I said.

Some people advocate consuming only water during a fast, but I think that's dangerous. I recommend drinking fruit and vegetable juices.

But I don't fast.

Very good. Then let's talk about your diet. Tell me what you have for breakfast every day.

I didn't want to tell him about the miller's bran: It wasn't high-value and tasted like sawdust. I thought it might beg questions about my mental health.

Two slices of whole-wheat bread and a banana, I said.

No butter, he said.

Of course not.

And lunch?

I didn't want to tell him it was just one green apple.

A tuna-fish sandwich, I said. I make it with yogurt instead of mayonnaise.

Plain nonfat yogurt, he said.

Of course.

That's good. And dinner?

Broccoli and tofu stir-fry, with bulgur instead of rice.

Excellent. And supplements?

You mean like protein powder?

I mean like vitamins and minerals.

I told him I didn't take anything like that and he said that might be why I was feeling less than optimal. He said it could be hard to get all your nutrients from food and that supplements could fill in the gaps. He said I should take separate supplements rather than a multivitamin, so as to increase absorption. He said the B-complex vitamins were particularly important, and vitamin C.

He said vitamin C was a stress vitamin, meaning it helped with stress, but also that it was used up more rapidly under stressful conditions. He said I should take it with every meal. He said Dr. Linus Pauling, the anti-nuclear activist and Nobel Laureate professor of chemistry at Stanford, said the optimum dose for most people was between 2,300 and 9,000 milligrams per day. He said Dr. Pauling had proven that vitamin C prevented the common cold, and that he himself could vouch for this, because he took 15,000 milligrams of vitamin C per day and hadn't had a cold in years. He said his body excreted whatever it couldn't use, and the only toxicity symptoms he'd ever experienced were loose stools and a slight burning during urination.

He took an index card out of his desk drawer and scribbled on it.

I'd like you to try my wheat-germ porridge for breakfast, he said. Two parts water, one part milk, and one part millet. Bring it all to a boil, then simmer for thirty minutes. It will still be a bit soupy. Stir in the wheat germ until you have the consistency of oatmeal. You can add cinnamon to taste.

14. October 1982

Nicole wanted to fix up her boss at the movie theater, Fiona Stewart, with my friend Aaron Goldman. Things hadn't worked out with the guy who'd sent Fiona flowers, and Nicole thought she and Aaron might get along since they were both native New Yorkers.

She suggested the four of us go out to dinner. I hadn't eaten in a restaurant for several months, and the prospect of doing so — of having to search for something on the menu that I could eat without triggering intense self-loathing — filled me with dread. But I felt I couldn't say no, because Fiona hated me and thought Nicole should break up with me. And while I could've lived with that, I was worried that maybe Fiona didn't hate me as much as Nicole claimed. I wondered if Nicole was using Fiona as a trial balloon, to voice feelings she didn't feel comfortable expressing to me directly.

They chose a Thai restaurant in Tarzana. I said Aaron and I would meet them there.

I drove over to his place in Van Nuys to pick him up. It was the same apartment I'd shared with him during my brief stint in college, after answering his ad in the *Pennysaver.*

He was ten years older than me, but he looked younger, even though he'd lost most of his hair and was graying at the temples; somehow these changes made him look preternaturally boyish. The day we met he told me the main thing he needed was someone to take care of his cat — Zappa — when he was on the road. Everything else was gravy, he said. We shook hands.

He drove a van for a courier service, delivering paintings and prints to galleries and museums in California and Arizona and New Mexico. Once he went to Minnesota. Before he left he told me he was going *out West*. I think he said this because he still had that East Coast orientation. I reminded him that he was, in fact, driving east, but he wouldn't concede my point.

He was moving a lot of Dali lithographs at the time. He'd bought one himself and hung it in our kitchen. It was a picture of Don Quixote in front of the windmills. This was before the story broke about all the forged Dalis. Owning a Dali — or thinking you owned a Dali — still meant something.

Aaron had been a huge fan of Frank Zappa and had all of his records, even the bootlegs. He had hundreds of records, everything from Captain Beefheart to Captain & Tennille. He kept them on the floor in the living room, in alphabetical piles. Sometimes I'd pull out *Weasels Ripped My Flesh* and look at the cover. It had an illustration of a guy in a suit holding an electric razor that was actually a weasel. The animal was clawing and biting the guy's cheek, but the guy was still smiling.

I say Aaron *had been* a Zappa fan, because by the time I started rooming with him he'd stopped listening to music entirely. Once I tried to get him to listen to Eno with me, but he wouldn't do it.

I'm just not into music anymore, he said.

I don't understand, I said. How can you turn something like that off?

I didn't do it on purpose, he said.

All he cared about was the Mets. They'd started to put together the team that would beat Boston in the World Series and he could sense the gathering storm and was getting ready. He kept his mint-condition Mets cap on a Styrofoam mannequin head that sat on top of one of his speaker cabinets. He wouldn't bend the brim and he wouldn't pull it down to his ears for fear of stretching it. Which was why I was so surprised when he answered the door and was wearing it.

I think she'll appreciate this as a fellow New Yorker, he said.

When we got to the restaurant Nicole and Fiona were waiting for us, sitting in a booth in the back, next to a sculpture of the Buddha that doubled as a fountain. We slid in across from them and Fiona and Aaron shook hands.

The Mets, she said.

This year is our year, he said.

She studied the orange interlocking N and Y on his cap, as if she was wondering what was under it. I didn't know if Nicole had told her he was bald.

If he felt uncomfortable under her gaze, he didn't show it. Maybe it was because he found her attractive. What with her russet hair and coffee-colored freckles, how could he not? She looked like the kind of girl the name *Fiona* had been invented for. I could easily see her coming down from the Highlands, or up from the Lowlands, wearing a cape, bearing a basket of muffins for her neighbors.

When the waitress came I didn't know what to order. I had planned to get some kind of stir fry and deal with my self-loathing later, but in the end I couldn't go through with it.

You can come back to me, I said.

Fiona rolled her eyes.

I'll have the yellow curry with chicken, she said.

Same for me, Nicole said.

I'll have Pad Thai with pork and a Thai iced tea, Aaron said.

The waitress took their menus and turned to me.

That happened faster than I anticipated, I said.

Take your time, she said.

I'm wondering if it would be possible for the chef to steam some broccoli and a chicken breast.

I don't know if he can steam a chicken breast.

No. Of course. My apologies. I wasn't clear about that. I'd like the broccoli steamed. The chicken breast could be boiled or baked. Just not fried. And if he could remove the skin that would be great.

We don't have fried chicken.

No. I mean yes. I meant stir-fried. But I take your point, because you wouldn't stir-fry a chicken breast. That would be crazy.

She took my menu and returned to the kitchen.

You're quite the spectacle, Fiona said.

He's been having stomach problems, Nicole said.

It's just that I can't eat anything spicy, I said.

Whatever, Fiona said.

You're rude, Aaron said. Are you a Yankees fan or something?

Fiona looked daggers at him.

You should take off your baseball cap, she said. It's not polite to wear a hat indoors.

When the waitress brought us our food Aaron reached into his pocket, pulled out some packages of ketchup, tore them open with his teeth, and painted his Pad Thai red.

I wasn't surprised. I'd seen him put ketchup on everything. He had a dedicated drawer in his kitchen for all the condiment packages he collected when he was on the road. But Fiona was disgusted and asked him how he could do such a thing.

I just like it, he said.

I stared down at my dish. The chicken breast was forlorn — the broccoli hadn't filled out the plate as much as I'd hoped.

That looks delicious, Aaron said.

I laughed. And then, unfortunately, I expelled a flatus.

Restricting my eating had made me flatulent. It had thrown my digestion out of whack. My stomach was empty most of the time, but it kept producing acid, which made me salivate more, which made me swallow more, which meant

I was swallowing more air, which meant there was more gas in my lower intestine, which meant I had more flatus events, as I'd taken to calling them, since the word *fart* had always sounded uncouth to me. But I smelled as raunchy as hell.

If you're sick, go to the hospital, Aaron said.

He eats a lot of tuna fish, Nicole said.

I had a dream the other night, Fiona said. I was riding on the back of a dolphin. Every time he breached I threw my arms over my head and filled my lungs with air. When we went back under the water I held my breath. I saw all kinds of fish, and sea fans, and coral, and turtles and rays and sharks and manatees. And I realized I was the scout for this school of dolphins, that I was the one determining whether the passage was safe. We were swimming along when all of a sudden I saw a net and I let out this screeching sound. And then I woke up.

I took a bite of my chicken. It was cold and dry. I wished I could've put some ketchup on it, but I was afraid of Fiona's reaction.

Fiona interpreted her dream. She told us that tuna fishermen were killing hundreds of thousands of dolphins every year. We were shocked.

You shouldn't eat tuna, she said. Not until the fishing industry changes its practices.

I knew she was right, but I was fed up. I'd been holding in another flatus and decided to let it go, which made me laugh, which made me expel another flatus, and then another, and then another.

Fiona stood up and tugged at Nicole's sleeve.

Let's go, she said.

I could see Nicole debating her options, trying to decide her loyalties. She slid out of the booth.

I'll call you later, she said.

As I drove Aaron back to his apartment I expected him to ask me something about what I'd had for dinner, or hadn't had for dinner, or why I was so thin. Part of me wanted him to ask. But he didn't say a word.

15. November 1982

When I first started starving myself I ran laps at a high-school track, jogging for six miles, then running intervals for six miles. I'd sprint a quarter-mile and jog three-quarters of a mile, then sprint a quarter-mile and jog half a mile, then sprint a quarter-mile and jog a quarter-mile, then sprint a mile. It was joyless, grinding. I never experienced the endorphin rush Nicole had described.

When I was too weak to run I took up swimming. I went to the YMCA every night, just before closing, when the pool wasn't too crowded, and swam two miles until my fatigue got to me. I kept having to decrease my distance, but it wasn't enough, because I was losing control of my breathing, and it was throwing off my rhythm, especially on my flip turns. One night I went into a turn too late and I smacked my head against the side, and I was so disoriented, and in so much pain, that I couldn't tell which way was up, and swam to the bottom of the pool and looked up and saw the lifeguard standing over the side, refracted in the light, and I pushed myself to the surface.

I didn't realize it, but my body was entering a conservation state. My pulse had slowed. My blood pressure and body temperature had dropped. My body was consuming itself. First it would eat the fat. Then it would eat the muscle. Then it would eat the vital organs.

When I was too weak to swim I took up yoga. A man named Richard Hittleman had a program on public television called *Yoga for Health*, and I watched and followed along. He began each episode explaining the benefits of yoga. His voice was soothing, hypnotic.

The practice of yoga imparts to the student an acute awareness of the beauty and power inherent in the body, he said. The distinctions between what we usually conceive of as body, mind, and spirit gradually diminish, and there occurs a merging or unification of the seemingly diverse aspects of our being. The realization that we can indeed function as an integrated whole is extremely meaningful. It effects a profound change in every aspect of our life.

Hittleman had an assistant, a woman named Cheryl. He gave her instructions and she then demonstrated the posture.

Cheryl was bone-thin. She wore sheer tights and a leotard. She moved with the grace of a dancer, through a set that resembled a Japanese teahouse. Her face was serene, composed. Her physical discipline had refined her spirit.

One morning I began a headstand in the middle of the living room as Hittleman guided me through each step.

Place a small pillow or a folded mat beneath your head, he said. Sit on your heels. Interlace your fingers and place your arms on the floor. Rest the top of your head on the mat. Cradle the back of your head in your clasped hands. Place your toes on the floor and push up so that your body forms an arch. Walk forward on your toes and move your knees as close to your chest as possible. Push off the floor lightly with your toes and transfer your weight so that it's evenly distributed between your head and forearms. Begin to straighten your legs. Make certain you are secure and well-balanced. Keep your legs close together. Keep your body as straight as possible. Breathe your yoga breath.

As I straightened my legs I felt the blood rushing to my head, swelling at my temples. I closed my eyes. Hittleman's voice trailed off, giving way to the sound of an acoustic guitar, to a slow melody I recognized from public-service announcements about smoking and air pollution that ran on television when I was a child. Somewhere in the midst of this nostalgia, and the tremendous silence between each note, I lost my balance and fell straight back, passing out before my feet hit the floor.

16. December 1982

When I went for my annual exam my doctor was alarmed. I'd weighed 145 pounds the year before; I now weighed 95. He immediately made an appointment for me to see an endocrinologist named Mikael Osheroff.

Dr. Osheroff took a series of measurements of my body in prone and standing positions. He poked at me with his fingers, pressed at the hollows in my limbs, measured their span with calipers. He told me I was an ectomorph, as if it were a diagnosis.

You might have a hormonal imbalance, he said. Or it could be a dysfunction in the satiety center of the hypothalamus, causing you to think you're full before you really are. Or lesions in the limbic system of your brain. Or an irregular output of vasopressin and gonadotropin. I can't be sure at this point. I'd like to admit you to the hospital and run some more tests. We'll start with a program of hormonal therapy. We'll give you injections twice a week to see if we can change the functioning of your brain.

I was stunned by the assumptions Dr. Osheroff was making, and how fast he was making them. The possibility that I had anorexia didn't occur to him; it couldn't occur to him. It wasn't how he saw the world.

I knew he was wrong, but he'd planted a seed of doubt. For the first time I wondered whether the starvation I'd thought was under my control ever really was. For the first time I wondered whether that sense of control was really my body tricking my mind.

The treatment plan he was proposing scared me. I was afraid if I went into the hospital under his care I'd never get out. When he excused himself to get some consent forms I got dressed and left.

17. January 1983

The *L.A. Times* ran a story about Marvin Kashner, Julia's doctor, and the eating-disorders program he directed at an area hospital. Nicole read the piece and wouldn't relent.

If you don't make an appointment I'm making one for you, she said.

He hasn't helped Julia, I said.

But you don't know how much worse it might have been.

And there's a teapot too small to be seen by a telescope that orbits the sun.

What is that supposed to mean?

It means I'm not seeing Kashner.

At my first session I explained to Kashner what the problem was.

I have a super-fast metabolism, I said. I eat something and I crap it right out.

It takes 36 hours to pass a meal, he said.

Not for me, I said.

He stared at me in disbelief. Then his beeper buzzed.

There's an emergency on the unit, he said. Please excuse me.

I sat there, alone, taking in the objects that filled his office, Indian artwork from all over the Southwest: a Hopi kachina, a Chumash basket, a Navajo rug. I waited half an hour before I realized he wasn't going to return.

When I told Nicole what had happened she begged me to give Kashner one more chance.

You can't treat this on your own, she said.

I didn't know what to say. There was nothing to treat, as far as I was concerned. I was fine. I was better than fine. But I loved her, and I didn't want her to get sick of me. I was terrified that she would break up with me. I had to find a way to string her along.

Maybe I could see a regular therapist, I said.

You need to see an expert, she said.

She accompanied me to my next appointment and sat in the lobby of the hospital's east wing, reading fashion magazines while I met with Kashner. But the same thing happened during the second session: He got a message on his beeper, excused himself, and never came back.

I wanted to go straight home but Nicole refused. She went to the admissions desk to complain, and as I stood there waiting for her a group of women came out from behind a set of double doors. I recognized them right away by their skinny arms and their skinny necks, and by the way they carried themselves — that self-possession that bordered on arrogance. They passed through the lobby and disappeared through another set of doors, on their way to some special place, I thought, where there was group therapy, and brand-new exercise equipment, and healthy food.

Part Two:
The Anorexia Nervosa
of Franz Kafka

1. May 1994

Years after I recovered, *Newsweek* ran a story about male anorexia. I knew about it only because I was seeing a therapist who happened to specialize in eating disorders. That's not why I was seeing him and we rarely discussed what I'd experienced, but a reporter from our local paper, looking for a local angle on the *Newsweek* story, had contacted him to see if he had any male patients she could interview. He asked me if I would be willing to talk to her and I said no, that part of my life was private.

The incidence of anorexia in the United States — for men and women — had been declining, and the percentage of anorexics who were men had remained unchanged for at least as long as Hilde Bruch had been writing about the disease: Men still represented 10 percent of all sufferers. This might be why other national magazines didn't jump on the bandwagon: There was no natural audience for the story. Most men didn't want to read about men who were starving themselves, and neither did most women, as it turned out.

And that's the most interesting part of this, because women's magazines had been featuring stories about female anorexia for years.

I think the beginning of an explanation can be found at the end of the *Newsweek* piece. One of the men the reporter profiled mentioned that he had to check out of an inpatient program because the female patients were so hostile toward him that it was making his condition even worse. Unfortunately, the reporter didn't ask him any follow-up questions about it.

Maybe some of the women in this program had preexisting issues with men, things they couldn't talk about with a man present. But I think there was something else going on: They were displaying a territorial instinct. They knew that it was different for this man, that however much his problem with food might resemble theirs it could never be the same — and that he had no right to be there. There was a question implicit in their anger, and they already knew the answer: A man couldn't have anorexia.

2. August 1353

Histories of anorexia always begin in Siena, with a young girl named Catherine. She was on her way home from a visit to her sister's house when she had her first vision of Christ. He was in the sky, looking down at her, radiating a golden light.

She gave her life to Him that day. When she turned seventeen she entered a Dominican order and began fasting as a way to display her devotion. She felt like she was concentrating her spirit, distilling it to its purest essence. She felt like she was living in a different kind of atmosphere, like she was breathing a different kind of air.

She starved to death in 1380, at the age of 33. In 1461 she was canonized. Soon women around the world were following her example, starving themselves to attain holiness, if not sainthood.

The practice reached its height during the 16th century, when a woman who claimed to eat nothing, or only the most symbolic of foods — the juice of a currant brushed across her lips with a bird's feather once a week — could draw crowds from miles away, bringing notoriety and commerce to even the smallest village. Members of the clergy would gather round a woman's bed and observe her for days on end, until they were convinced the cause of her sustenance was truly divine.

In the 17th century the nature of fasting began to change. Women continued to starve themselves as a way to develop a kind of inwardness, a kind of spirituality, but it no longer took place under the auspices of a church. These new self-starvers were, in most cases, not affiliated with a particular faith: It was a private religion they were cultivating, a sense of mystery that had been missing from their lives.

American and European newspapers started featuring stories about these women, referring to them as *miraculous maidens* and rendering their images in before-and-after drawings — the before drawings in front view, the after drawings in profile, to accentuate the maiden's emaciation.

But these stories were more the stuff of scandal, and aroused skepticism rather than wonder.

Priests and pastors still gathered round the starving woman's bed. But they were joined now by doctors and medical researchers — men trained to begin every inquiry from a position of doubt — who poked the woman with instruments, examined her stool and urine, and weighed her every hour on the hour.

When they took a break in their surveillance, late at night, one of the maiden's loved ones — usually her mother, or her sister — would sneak in and give her some food, always at great risk, because if the doctors and medical researchers learned of the subterfuge they would initiate a round-the-clock vigil, until the maiden confessed that she'd been eating all along, or refused to confess, and died of starvation.

3. October 1873

The English physician Sir William Gull and the French neurologist Charles Lasegue were the first to identify and treat self-starvation as a medical condition. They did so entirely independent of each other, and, upon learning of the other's work, rushed to claim credit for discovering the new disease.

Lasegue called the condition he observed *l'anorexie hysterique*. He viewed it as fundamentally psychological in nature, and spent much of his time considering the patient's relationships with her family members before making his diagnosis.

Male physicians had long used the term *hysteros* — the Greek word for uterus — to designate diseases that were thought to afflict only women. Designating a disease as a form of hysteria both minimized its severity and marginalized it as something peculiar and particular to women. It reinforced the myth that women were irrational and needed to be cared for by men. In writing about a patient who wound a rose-colored ribbon around her waist every morning, never letting herself exceed its measure, Lasegue conjectured that the knot in the ribbon represented something knotted in her uterus, in that great empty space inside her.

Gull first referred to anorexia as *apepsia hysterica*, but he didn't want to talk about emotions or engage in metaphors; he saw the disease as a purely physiological dysfunction, treatable only through diet and medication. His approach allowed for a possibility he never considered and perhaps never would've entertained: If anorexia was a physical rather than a psychological disorder, then it could afflict men as well as women.

4. June 1880

The first hunger artists appeared in Europe and the United States at the end of the 19th century. Other than the fact that they were all men, there wasn't a substantive difference between them and the fasting women of the previous two centuries, who had gradually, with varying degrees of calculation and success, turned their starvation into profit.

But maybe gender made all the difference. The miraculous maidens were secretive about their reasons for starving and tried to create the illusion they'd gone without food for years and years. They never left the confines of their bedrooms, instead surrounding themselves with friends and family, letting their mothers or sisters regulate their spectacle.

The hunger artists, by contrast, were up front about the fact that they were trying to make money. Many of them had managers to promote them, to book them into the largest public venues possible. Sensitive to the whims of the marketplace, they limited the length of their fasts: Long enough to build suspense, but short enough to keep people's interest. Forty days was optimal: the exact length of time the prophets of Jewish and Christian scripture — Moses, Elijah, Jesus — went into the desert and denied themselves food.

The first hunger artist was a physician from England named Henry Tanner. As a young man Tanner had gone several days without food due to an illness and discovered he felt better than ever. He believed his accidental fast had given him access to a secret, spiritual force that could not only preserve his strength but increase it. In 1848 he went to the United States and began practicing medicine in Minneapolis, lecturing his patients on the virtues of temperance and prescribing fasts as a cure for certain diseases.

In 1880 he heard about the "Brooklyn Enigma," a woman named Mollie Fancher who claimed she'd gone years without eating. Fancher had reached such a level of celebrity that the renowned physician William Hammond had asked if he could observe her to verify the truth of her claims. But she'd refused — for the sake of propriety, she said.

On learning of this, Tanner wrote to Hammond and volunteered himself for observation. But he lacked Fancher's fame and Hammond wasn't interested. Neither was anyone else, for that matter. So Tanner moved to New York City and set himself up in Clarendon Hall in the East Village and began a fast for forty days.

People paid twenty-five cents a head to view Tanner kneeling on an empty stage, his body backlit during the evening hours to accentuate his increasing emaciation. Soon he was receiving fan mail, upwards of a hundred letters a day, including one much-publicized missive from Mollie Fancher herself, the contents of which he would not reveal. Women serenaded him on the street. Men renamed their football clubs in his honor. The Brooklyn Museum even offered to stuff his body and put him on display should he die during the fast.

By the 11th day the medical community caved in. The newspaper coverage had become so sensational that a team of prominent doctors asked if they could set themselves up in Clarendon Hall to monitor him.

On the 40th day Tanner broke his fast, a crowd of two thousand standing rapt as he ate a quarter of a peach, devoured a giant Georgia watermelon, and drank a glass of rice milk in a single gulp. When he finished off half a pound of broiled beefsteak and half a pound of sirloin they burst into wild applause.

But his success was his undoing. When the *New York Times* reported that Clarendon Hall had cleared almost $3,000 from Tanner's "stunt," the medical establishment turned against him, dismissing his experiment as a circus sideshow. They pointed to those first 11 days, when no one had monitored him. They noted how he'd gone out for haircuts and photo shoots and walks through Washington Square, all opportune times for him to sneak a bit of food. And while it was true he'd lost 40 pounds, he'd held up well all things considered, far better than possible if he'd truly been starving himself.

Feeling defeated, Tanner faded into obscurity, having lost the true object of his quest: scientific proof of the benefits of fasting. But he'd inadvertently spawned the next entertainment craze.

The hunger artists who imitated Tanner always began their fasts by claiming they would best his performance. But it was difficult to do, and several of them died trying.

The risk of death only whetted the public's appetite. Doctors began hiring themselves out as official witnesses, knowing their presence would confer legitimacy to the hunger artist's fast. They'd record his weight, draw his blood, check his pulse and breathing, and collect samples of his urine and stool. When asked why they were participating they always said the same thing: It was an opportunity to study the effects of starvation on real human subjects, rather than extrapolating from experiments on animals.

The popularity of hunger art reached its peak in 1895, when there were over 200 known practitioners. It had a revival during the 1920s, but it was brief. Even in Berlin, where the art of fasting had been most popular, the cultural climate was changing. As National Socialism became a force in Germany the hunger artists were banned from performing. The Nazis viewed them as *untermenschen*, vermin, the weakness that was corrupting the state. But it was the rise of cinema, the new spectacle destined to replace all forms of theater, that truly signaled their end. By 1930 they had all but disappeared.

5. May 1922

Franz Kafka had read about the hunger artists in the Prague dailies when he was a boy. Their stories made a deep impression on him, in particular the story of a hunger artist in Berlin who conducted his fasts in a neighborhood steakhouse. The man would set himself up in a glass box in the middle of the dining room and watch as patrons gorged themselves on rare beef and red wine, utterly indifferent to him.

Kafka wrote "A Hunger Artist" two years before he died. In it he chronicles the demise of hunger art through the story of one hunger artist who refuses to quit, who keeps practicing his craft long after the public has lost interest. Kafka remains faithful to the historical record for the most part, rendering both the mundane and grotesque details of the hunger artist's life: the cage he imprisons himself in during his fast, the black tights he wears to exaggerate his emaciation, the attending physicians in their starched white coats, the pretty young women who help him out of his cage when he breaks his fast, so repulsed by the sight of him that they burst into tears.

Kafka's hunger artist, like all of his characters, is blinded by reason, by an extreme form of logic. It leads him to do things that are self-destructive. It makes him a mystery to himself, and to us. At the end of the story he explains his behavior to the overseer of a group of workers who have come to clean out his cage:

"I always wanted you to admire my fasting," said the hunger artist. "We do admire it," said the overseer, affably. "But you shouldn't admire it," said the hunger artist. "Well then we don't admire it," said the overseer, "but why shouldn't we admire it?" "Because I have to fast, I can't help it," said the hunger artist. "What a fellow you are," said the overseer, "and why can't you help it?" "Because," said the hunger artist, lifting his head a little and speaking, with his lips pursed, as if for a kiss, right into the overseer's ear, so that no syllable might be lost, "because I couldn't find the food I liked. If I had found it, believe me, I should have made no fuss and stuffed myself like you or anyone else."

These are his last words. The men bury him and put a panther in his place. Soon there are people gathering around the panther the way they once did the hunger artist, mesmerized by the great cat pacing back and forth, its every movement a show of strength and vitality.

I'd been fasting for six months when I first read "A Hunger Artist." I wanted to read it because of the title — I thought it would reveal something to me about what I was experiencing. I had no idea Kafka was documenting a historical phenomenon. The story was just as indeterminate and disturbing to me as everything else I'd read by Kafka, so I just assumed he'd invented it.

The German psychiatrist Manfred Fichter diagnosed Kafka with anorexia nervosa in an article he wrote for the *International Journal of Eating Disorders* in 1987. Drawing on Kafka's stories, letters, and diaries, Fichter summarized his findings as follows:

1. Kafka was thin.
2. Kafka wrote about food and eating.
3. Kafka had an ascetic personality.
4. Kafka had sadomasochistic fantasies.
5. Kafka was depressed and compulsive.
6. Kafka was achievement oriented.
7. Kafka never individuated from his parents. He feared and hated his father, who was big and strong, and loved his mother, who was controlling.
8. Kafka was sexually repressed.
9. Kafka didn't see himself as a real man.

Fichter's argument goes something like this:

1. People with anorexia have a certain personality type.
2. Kafka had this personality type.
3. Therefore, Kafka had anorexia.

The argument relies on two false suppositions:

1. All people with anorexia have a certain personality type.
2. All people who have this personality type have anorexia.

Fichter's argument isn't valid, but it doesn't need it to be. To generate academic discussion and debate it just has to look and sound like logic.

Other writers have referenced these same personality traits to argue that Kafka was gay (when being gay was considered a mental illness), that he had schizoid personality disorder, and that he had borderline personality disorder.

I can't pretend to understand this desire to diagnose a historical figure in this way, particularly when it's a writer like Kafka, whose method *was* metaphor. It was how he distilled his experience, not just in his stories, but in his letters and his diaries as well. He didn't use figures of speech to achieve particular effects; he used figures of speech because, for him, all language was figurative. That's why his stories are so unsettling, so unresolved. Like truly troubling dreams, they're closed systems, private, impenetrable. I might interpret "A Hunger Artist" as a parable, Kafka commenting on the alienation of the artist in an industrialized society through the depiction of an actual starving artist, a man whose art is art for art's sake, something he does out of a sense of vocation. Or I might understand the end of the story as a form of foreshadowing, the hunger artist as the Jew and the panther as the Nazi who, holding the world in his thrall, will eradicate the Jew, erase him from the face of the earth. But these interpretations don't tell me anything objective about the story.

A metaphor that has a definite, singular meaning is simply a shitty metaphor. And that's the problem with Fichter: To make his diagnosis, he has to interpret Kafka's writing — and the historical phenomenon he was writing about — in a very narrow, literal way. So hunger art corresponds to anorexia: *That's what it really is.* But the past isn't a metaphor for the present. The past isn't a metaphor for anything.

The hunger artist dies because he exceeds the forty days prescribed to him, because he goes too long without eating. But that's not really why he dies. He dies because people stop watching him. His life, like all of ours, is contingent upon being seen.

Kafka understood this. That's the only conclusion I feel comfortable drawing from the story.

Self-starvation is a performance with a paradox, because the same thing that makes you visible makes you invisible. By disappearing you appear, and by appearing you disappear.

6. May 1923

Fasting was a sanctioned legal procedure in pre-Christian Ireland, a way for one man to seek restitution from another without resorting to violence. The injured party would go to the offender's home and sit on his doorstep and fast until he was compensated for his damages. This typically took no longer than a day, because the offender faced tremendous public shame and ostracization if he didn't comply.

Over time fasting became a protest strategy, but its use was rare and reserved for men, until the British suffragettes started using the practice in the early 20th century.

The suffragettes called their fasts *hunger strikes*. Marion Dunlop was the first to do it, when she was imprisoned in 1909. The British authorities, fearing she would become a martyr, immediately released her from the Holloway Gaol, and she was able to avoid force-feeding. But the women who followed her weren't so fortunate.

Between 1909 and 1914 almost 200 British suffragettes endured brutal force-feeding in prison. Many suffered it multiple times. But they were forging a powerful protest procedure. They would demonstrate, get arrested, go on a hunger strike, and endure force-feeding. When they were released from prison, they would go to the press with their stories, describing, in graphic detail, what they had experienced. Their accounts were harrowing to read and helped build support for the suffragette cause.

Inspired by Marion Dunlop, Lady Constance Lytton, a member of the British aristocracy, began working for women's suffrage in the fall of 1909. She marched with her fellow suffragettes and engaged in the exact same forms of civil disobedience as they did, but, because of her social status, she received special treatment from law enforcement. She literally couldn't get arrested until she threw a rock at the Chancellor of the Exchequer's Rolls-Royce Silver Ghost.

Her special treatment continued in prison. She spent one night in a cell in Holloway Gaol's first division — the section for political prisoners — listening to the screams of her sisters who were being force fed in the second division, the section for common criminals. The next day she was moved to the infirmary, examined by the medical staff, and released.

Things continued in this way for six months. Lytton threw rocks at cars, got arrested, then received special treatment at Holloway. Determined to overcome the privileges of her class, to experience the same degree of suffering as her comrades, she cut her hair, started wearing loose-fitting clothes and pince-nez glasses, and changed her name to Miss Jane Warton. She attended a demonstration in Liverpool, where no one knew her, threw a rock at a member of Parliament's car, was arrested, sent to the second division at Walton Gaol, went on a hunger strike, and was force-fed eight times. When she was released she had a heart attack and a series of strokes that eventually led to her death.

Just as some writers see hunger art as anorexia in disguise, some see anorexia as a hunger strike in disguise. They argue that while the two appear to occupy different cultural spheres — one private, playing out before family and friends, and the other public, performed before a large, mostly anonymous audience — both are, in fact, struggles for control, for ownership of the body. Both are forms of resistance. Both are expressions of anger.

In this sense, the only real difference between anorexia and a hunger strike is who gets to name the behavior: The hunger striker declares the meaning of her fast so people know how to interpret it, while the anorexic doesn't say anything about what she's doing, so other people — friends, family, doctors — tell her.

It's this passiveness, or passive-aggressiveness, that's so unsettling. It's troubling to think that suffragettes put their lives on the line only to have their granddaughters and great-granddaughters starve themselves in silence, for private, personal reasons, rather than a greater cause, a greater good. It's troubling to think that a woman would turn her anger against herself, against her body, rather than directing it outward. And that's the real motivation for recasting anorexia as a hunger strike: It's an attempt to locate anorexia within the history of feminism, to resolve those aspects of the disease that seem so regressive.

7. May 1982

Hilde Bruch first used the term *me-too anorexic* during a lecture at George Washington University that formed the basis for "Four Decades of Eating Disorders," an article she contributed to *The Handbook of Psychotherapy for Anorexia Nervosa and Bulimia*, published in 1985, just after she died.

> *The patients who were seen during the 1950s and 1960s had in common that each one was an original inventor of this effort at self-assertion.... They had never heard about such a condition, nor had their parents or even their physicians. Yet they shared certain reactions – particularly the conviction that they were not sick, but, on the contrary, were doing something positive about their lives.... At no time did I have reason to doubt the genuineness of their symptoms and reactions.*

> *This originality gave to the behavior of each individual patient an aura of special power and superhuman discipline. Some changes seem to have occurred when anorexia nervosa became more frequent. Those who developed the illness during the 1970s often had 'known' about the illness, or even knew someone who had it. During the past few years several patients deliberately 'tried it out' after having*

watched a TV program or having assembled a science project. There is no doubt in my mind that this 'me-too' picture is associated with changes in the clinical − in particular, the psychological − picture; I am not yet able to define them, except that something like 'passion' has gone out of the picture. Instead of the fierce search for independence, these new 'me-too' anorexics compete with or cling to each other. That they seek support in self-help groups or respond to the various 'programs' that have sprung up all over the country may be an illustration of this development. The desire to be special, unique, or extraordinary is expressed with less vigor and urgency, and I cannot suppress the suspicion that in some the symptoms are imitative or faked. It is my feeling that ultimately the condition will lose its specific psychodynamic meaning. As it becomes more commonplace, the picture will become blurred and gradually disappear until the conditions are right again for genuine primary anorexia nervosa.

The lecture was an occasion for Bruch to look back on her career, and for her peers to celebrate her. But it prompted her to engage in a troubling kind of nostalgia.

The contrast she draws is startling. She admired the women she treated in the 1950s and 1960s. She held them in high regard. She sympathized with them. They had *an aura of special power*. Their anorexia was *genuine*.

She didn't anticipate the impact of popular culture. But it's almost as if she wanted the conditions to be right again, wants to return to the cultural moment when she first identified fasting as a disease.

Because while William Gull and Charles Lasegue gave anorexia nervosa its name, Hilde Bruch determined its meaning. Hilde Bruch invented anorexia nervosa.

Bruch was born in Germany in 1904 to a middle-class Jewish family. She went into medicine because it was one of the few professions open to Jews at the time, but fled the country in 1933 after the Nazis shut down her pediatric practice.

She arrived in the United States the following year. With much effort she was able to bring most of her family over before the war began, but she lost her older sister, Hannah, and her younger brother, Michael, to the camps.

She never married and never had children. Her family described her as strong-willed, irritable, and sensitive to slights. In 1937 she was placed in the psychiatric unit of Columbia Hospital in New York City after attempting suicide. The treatment she received sparked her professional interest in psychoanalysis and informed the methods she later developed for the diagnosis and treatment of anorexia.

The media accelerated the transmission of anorexia exponentially in the 1970s and it made Bruch bristle. She'd long argued that anorexia had its origins in the nursing behaviors of the mother − in the harmful ways a mother granted, or didn't grant, food to her infant daughter. Bruch believed that these behaviors persisted in other forms as the daughter grew into adulthood, eventually leading the daughter to starve herself in retaliation.

It's almost as if Bruch feared losing her own sense of specialness. The specialness she felt in having discovered these women when no one else knew who or what they were. The specialness she felt in having dedicated her entire career to describing them and helping them. She couldn't acknowledge that there had always been a social dimension to the disease, that family wasn't the only crucible, nor psychoanalysis the only treatment. She couldn't recognize the role her own work had played in sensationalizing anorexia, in packaging it for popular consumption, in paving the way for a series of confessional memoirs and television movies.

Instead she predicted the end of anorexia, imagined its gradual disappearance and eventual reemergence at some point in the future, when, once again, it might serve as a way for women to feel unique.

If I had anorexia I caught it from Julia — who had it — and Nicole — who didn't. But my experience of the disease wasn't different by virtue of this.

It's impossible to separate the physiological effects of starvation from the psychological effects. The lack of food distorts your thinking. You starve yourself in part as a way to cope with the feelings brought on by starving yourself. The only way out is for you to eat. If you eat more your thinking will begin to change. If you eat more you will want to continue eating more. But this is precisely what you cannot do, because just as eating makes you hungry, starving makes you want to starve. The less you eat the less you want to eat.

Bruch's *me-too anorexics* may have had programs where they could "cling" to each other, but sooner or later their hunger was going to catch up to them. Sooner or later their hunger was going to make them behave just like the women she had treated earlier in her career, the women she had deemed worthy of her sympathy, and her admiration.

8. February 1983

Nicole was worried about Julia, but it was more than that: Her feelings about Julia were mixed up with her ideas about beauty, with her insecurities about her own appearance. She always compared herself to other women.

When we were in line at a supermarket checkout she'd flip through the pages of fashion magazines and show me photos of the anorexic models. Their beauty was assertive, severe.

Look at her, Nicole would say. Her thighs are no bigger than her calves.

When Karen Carpenter died these magazines started running cover stories about anorexia nervosa all the time. But as well-intentioned as the stories were, they always suffered from the advertising that surrounded them, from the tension between selling anorexia and educating women about it.

Part Three:
The Land of Enchantment

1. June 1981

The idea of going to Mexico began in an art history class, a survey of the modern period from neoclassicism to the present. The professor was a long-haired Englishman named Taylor. He stood on a stage in a five hundred-seat lecture hall, in sandals and jeans and a brightly colored dashiki, and showed us slides of famous paintings, the images projected onto a large white screen behind him.

Each painting had a story, some sort of intrigue Taylor would elaborate, either about its commission, or its reception, or its revolutionary technique. Once he had given us a sense of the social and economic forces at work at the time of the painting's production he'd segue and connect the moment of the painting to the present, to crimes and atrocities I knew little or nothing about. For his lecture on *The Third of May 1808* he talked about the ways Goya had broken from the heroic tradition in Spanish painting, then jumped to a series of prints from *The Disasters of War*, juxtaposing them with black-and-white photos of civilians who had been tortured and murdered in El Salvador.

On the final day of class a hunched man in an ill-fitting gray suit shuffled onto the stage and told us he'd be giving the final lecture in place of Professor Taylor, who had taken ill. This stand-in professor then proceeded to give a dull treatise on Monet's use of blue, laced with asides about Professor Taylor, who, he maintained, was unfit for academia, making it clear to anyone who may have doubted it that this was in fact Professor Taylor, pretending to be one of his peers.

Taylor had been railing against his colleagues all semester long, condemning them for their conformist, careerist ambitions, their little articles in their little journals, their little conferences where they debated for hours and hours about the thread count in 15th-century Flemish tapestries. The tyranny of the scholar, he called it, and now he was acting it out, until, about 20 minutes into his impersonation, his voice began to change, to pick up some of the patter and music of British English, and he gradually stood straighter, and took on more and more of the mannerisms we'd come to know him by, and the timbre of his voice was fully restored, and he peeled off his shabby professorial clothes and became Professor Taylor again, standing in front of us like some hippie superman.

There's an FBI agent with us today, he said. They've had me under surveillance for a long time. They want me to shut my mouth. They want me to teach this class the way it's taught in every other university in the country, to give you a copy of Janson's *History of Art* and quiz you on it once a week. They want me to teach you about Pop Art and Minimalism and environmental sculpture instead of the work of the Cuban muralists and the billboard artists of Nicaragua. But I don't care. They can keep on harassing me. They can try and have me deported. They can try and have me killed. I'm still going to say what I have to say.

When he walked off the stage everyone in the auditorium stood and cheered, myself included. But I found it a disquieting moment, seeing this man I'd admired the whole semester now being adulated like a rock star. There was something self-promoting about it, a cult of personality he was encouraging that made me uncomfortable. I looked around me, wondering whether I was the only one who felt this way, suddenly alienated, suddenly paranoid at the thought of an FBI agent in the room. But if anyone else felt what I was feeling I couldn't see it in their faces. For a moment I wondered whether the FBI agent was me.

A couple of days later I was walking through a campus food court and stopped to talk to a soft-spoken man with a long beard and a ponytail. He was selling copies of a magazine put out by the North American Congress on Latin America. We talked for a while and then he told me about a group called the Network in Solidarity with the People of Guatemala that was having a meeting that evening. He said I was welcome to come. I hesitated. I'd never been an activist and had an inveterate fear of groups, but Professor Taylor had made me feel like I needed to do something, so I said I would go.

About ten of us sat on the floor of an empty classroom at the south end of campus and listened to a reporter from the *L.A. Times* describe a massacre that had just taken place in the village of El Arbolito, in the department of Petén. A few Guatemalan soldiers had entered the village and spray-painted a left-wing slogan on the side of the elementary school. The next day four army platoons rounded up all the residents and marched them at gunpoint onto the school soccer field. They pulled 47 men from the crowd and, one by one, accused each man of having painted the slogan.

Then they beat each man, hooded him, gassed him, burned him, and shot him as his loved ones were forced to watch.

These kinds of massacres were happening almost every day, the reporter said. The Guatemalan government, with the support of the Reagan administration, was systematically murdering the country's Indigenous population, the descendants of the Maya.

2. May 1982

I began listening to KPFK for Irving Pitkin, and Alan Watts' lectures on Zen, but as I became more involved with the Network in Solidarity with the People of Guatemala, I started tuning in to the station's news and public affairs programming. It felt like attending one of Professor Taylor's lectures: painful, but necessary. KPFK reported stories no one else wanted to talk about.

But it distanced me even further from Nicole. I was at her apartment one night, watching the network news, when General Efrain Rios Montt, the newest dictator of Guatemala, appeared on screen in military dress. He said he was praying to Lord Jesus Christ to bring peace to the hearts and minds of the Guatemalan people, but that subversives should know he was ready to use weapons to fulfill his Christian duty, and that he would execute anyone who acted against the government. Then the network reporter came on screen, and, in an effort to provide more context, said U.S. government officials had spoken with him on the condition of anonymity and told him that, while they acknowledged abuses on the part of the Guatemalan military, such brutal tactics were needed to root out the communist guerrillas who were hiding among the Guatemalan Indians.

This guy's such a prick, I said.

I don't like it when you talk like that, Nicole said.

But it's fucking horseshit.

Maybe there are two sides to it.

I couldn't tell if she really believed what she was saying or was just saying it to try to separate herself from my anger, to preserve something essential about herself. And I didn't care.

You don't know what the fuck you're talking about, I said.

She went to her bedroom and the story on the television changed. Now, instead of Rios Montt, there were images of Ronald Reagan visiting a farm in Iowa, posing for pictures with a giant pig.

I showed up at KPFK on a Saturday afternoon, hoping to speak with someone about volunteering. There was no one in the reception area, so I walked around the station until I saw a guy in one of the studios. He had a bowl haircut and big aviator glasses. He waved me in and introduced himself.

I'm Mike Rushmore, he said.

I was starstruck. Mike Rushmore did the evening news. He was my Edward R. Murrow, my Walter Cronkite. I told him I wanted to volunteer and he asked me if I had a background in journalism. I was about to say no and tell him that I was thinking more of stuffing envelopes or something like that. But then I remembered in junior high I'd been a reporter for my school newspaper and had learned about the inverted pyramid and *who, what, where, when, why* and *how.*

I've done a little bit, I said.

Because I need someone to write copy for me, he said.

I started working for Mike the following Saturday. He had me stand at the teleprinter and check the AP and the UPI feeds for minor stories, filler pieces he could insert at the end of the broadcast in case he finished the main stories earlier than he anticipated. I found it stressful, because stories were spooling off the teleprinter constantly, and I had to make a quick decision, operate on a hunch, an instinct about what Mike would like. Once I tore a story off the feed there would be no time to go back and choose something else — I had to commit to it, because it was going to take me time to work it up into something Mike could read on air.

Either I got lucky that first day or Mike was being nice to me, because it was the only time he ever used something I wrote. I picked a story about proposed changes to CAFE standards for U.S. automobiles and turned it into a multi-paragraph essay I felt really good about, but when I gave it to him he frowned.

This isn't a novel, he said. You've got to get in and get out.

I cut it down and gave it back to him and he frowned again.

It's still too much detail, he said. Don't get so attached to certain words.

We went back and forth like this for hours. Mike was exasperated. Finally he took out his pen and drew black lines through almost everything I'd written, then went on air. But he read it — all two sentences of it — and I felt so proud.

3. July 1982

The Guatemalan army entered San Francisco Nentón, in the department of Huehuetenango, rounded up all the residents, and marched them at gunpoint into the village church. They took the women out in groups, back to their homes, raped them, and cut off their heads with machetes. They went back for the children, took them into the coffee fields, threw them into the air, and stabbed them with bayonets. They went back for the men, led them into the street, tied their hands behind their backs, cut off their ears, gouged out their eyes, burned them with blowtorches, peeled off their skin, and shot each of them in the back of the head. They carried all 376 bodies back to the church and set it on fire.

The American newspapers didn't report the massacre in San Francisco Nentón. The Network in Solidarity with the People of Guatemala learned of it through a sister organization in Mexico City and decided to hold a candlelight vigil.

About 300 of us gathered at the Veterans' Cemetery and marched down Sepulveda Boulevard, crossed Wilshire, and formed a line on the sidewalk in front of the Federal Building. Most cars just raced past us, but occasionally someone would honk, or roll down their window and call us communists.

A man in a Castro cap walked up and down the line, thanked us for coming out, and gave us new candles as we needed them. I recognized him from the Network meetings — he was usually the one who introduced a speaker, or set up the projector or the PA system, or talked to the reporters from Pacifica. At the end of the vigil he told us there would be a demonstration the next day, in case any of us could attend. He said the Casa Nicaragua would be providing food.

I called Mr. Cox and told him I was sick and got to the Federal Building at 8 a.m. A few Network members had already drawn outlines of bodies on the front steps and written a statistic inside each one: the number of Guatemalans who had been murdered since the war began (150,000); the number of CIA operatives in the country (54); the amount of U.S. money being funneled through Israel to purchase the Galil rifles that were being used to kill the Indians ($500,000 a day). As government employees started arriving for work they were polite, and stepped over the bodies, but none of them stopped to read the statistics.

When more people arrived we made signs that said *Stop the Genocide in Guatemala* and *Reagan Is a War Criminal*. We formed a line on the sidewalk again and the man in the Castro cap walked up and down, but this time he had a guitar, and he played songs by Silvio Rodriguez, and we sang along. *Vamos a andar. Para llegar. A la vida.*

By midday I was dizzy. The exterior of the Federal Building was covered with concrete fins that shaded the offices inside, that made the windows shimmer in the heat, and I thought the building was a mirage, a phantom that was about to disappear. I sat down on the sidewalk and tried to steady myself. I closed my eyes to let my hunger settle, but I couldn't stop the white spots flashing in my head. The man in the Castro cap approached me and asked if I was okay.

You should get something to eat, he said.

The Casa Nicaragua had set up card tables with trays of rice and beans and fried plantains, but these were foods I'd already eliminated from my diet.

I just need a minute, I said.

I hated the fact that I had to eat. I hated the fact that to go on living, I had to take these objects outside my body and put them inside my body. It was exhausting. I was sick of it. I didn't want to do it anymore.

As I think about it now I wonder what would have happened if, instead of holding a sign and singing with the other protesters, I had gone to the front steps of the Federal Building and declared a hunger strike. Maybe it would have changed everything. Maybe it would have changed nothing.

That afternoon Ed Asner showed up to lend his support. Asner was something of a hero to me. I'd grown up watching him on the *Mary Tyler Moore Show*, and then on

Lou Grant, which CBS had just canceled even though the ratings were good. The network wouldn't give him an explanation, but he suspected it was because of his involvement in the Central America Solidarity Movement. He was the president of the Screen Actors Guild at this time and was getting a lot of grief from former Guild president Charlton Heston, a Reagan crony who, like Reagan three decades earlier, was accusing fellow actors of being traitors and communists.

Asner stood on the steps of the Federal Building and talked about the growing refugee crisis in the Mexican state of Chiapas. Over 100,000 Guatemalans had crossed the border and were living in squalid makeshift camps, and the Mexican government was going to start repatriating them at the end of the month. If that happened, he said, they would face certain death.

4. April 1983

Nicole didn't want me to go to Mexico. She said it was dangerous. I wasn't sure if she meant it was dangerous for everyone, or just dangerous for me, and didn't ask. I was determined to go and didn't want to fight with her.

So that's it, she said. You're just going to leave and never come back?

No, I said. I don't know.

I don't see how you can make a decision like this without talking to me.

This isn't about us.

Of course it is.

I need to do something, I said.

You are doing something. You can do more if you want. But you need to stay here.

I felt bad submitting my resignation at work. Mr. Cox had gone to some lengths to create a new position for me, and I could see he was disappointed.

I thought you and I were in this for the long haul, he said.

I'm really grateful to you, sir, I said.

I saw you moving into management at some point. After the dust had settled on your stator failures, of course.

It's been an honor working with you, sir.

Those last few days were long. Most of my deliveries were in San Fernando and I finished them early, but instead of going back to the shop I drove into the San Gabriel Mountains and parked. It would be smog season soon, but for now the sky was clear, and blue, and I could see for miles. I understood why the Spanish, looking south at this valley that was really a desert, had built a mission here, in San Fernando, instead of on the other side the valley, the side they always showed in the movies, looking north from Mulholland Drive.

Nicole gave me a going-away present the night before I left, a guidebook to Mexico called *The Land of Enchantment*. It had a picture of Chichen Itza on the cover.

In case you want to do some sightseeing, she said.

I kissed her. It was a thank-you kiss at first, but then I kept going, because I thought I should, because I thought that's what people did before an extended separation, to give their time apart its proper significance, to imprint the memory of their bodies on each other. I was trying to remember the feelings I'd once felt, but she pulled away.

I can't do this, she said.

It had been months since we'd made love. I thought it was because I'd transcended the needs of my body. I didn't realize my loss of desire was a physiological response to my starvation.

My skin had turned yellow. The blonde hair that once covered my arms and legs had receded into something finer, white. My veins were blue at my wrists. My hipbones stuck out like the wings of a bird. And yet I thought I was still attractive to her. I thought my starving had made her want me even more, even if I no longer wanted her.

I don't feel that way, she said.

I asked her when her feelings had changed, but she didn't know. And then I felt a nausea come over me that I couldn't relieve, because there was nothing inside me to throw up.

5. May 1983

I took a plane to Mexico City, a plane to Tuxtla Gutiérrez, and a bus to San Cristobal. I arrived after midnight and checked into a cheap hotel. The room was small and cold. There was a painting of a woman in a blue tunic above the bed. I unpacked my bag, lay down, and read the introduction to the guidebook until I fell asleep.

In Mexico City, in the district of Popotla, you will find the remains of a giant bald cypress tree. Neighborhood residents set it on fire many times over the years, and in the winter of 1980 they finally burned it to the ground.

This was the tree where Cortés rested the morning after the night he escaped from Tenochtitlan, before he rode on to Tlaxcala, put together a new army, returned to Tenochtitlan, blockaded the city, cut off its water supply, and destroyed the Aztec empire.

He'd arrived in Tenochtitlan six months earlier, with 1,000 Spanish soldiers in tow. He knew he had to proceed with caution – Tenochtitlan was a highly developed city-state,

with a powerful military. So he met with the Aztec king —
Moctezuma — ingratiated himself, and bided his time.

When he was certain he had Moctezuma's complete trust he
and his men killed him, raided his palace, and looted it of all
its gold. Upon learning this, the Aztec military razed the
bridges over the network of canals surrounding the palace
so that Cortés and his men couldn't get away. They holed
up for eight days, and on the ninth day, running out of
food, Cortés sent a communiqué to the commander of the
Aztec military requesting safe passage. He promised to leave
behind all the gold, though this was another bluff, because
his real plan was to escape that night using a portable
bridge his men had built.

They left the palace after sunset and reached the first canal
without resistance. They thought they were in the clear
until sentries sounded the alarm and the Aztec military
stormed the causeway. Most of Cortés' men jumped into the
canal and tried to swim to the opposite bank, but were so
weighed down by the gold they'd strapped to their bodies
that they drowned. But Cortés survived and cleared the last
canal, and the Aztecs, believing they'd defeated him once
and for all, gave up the chase.

Bernal Diaz de Castillo, a captain in Cortés' army, also made it out alive, and he described this night, and everything that led up to it, in his first-person chronicle, The True History of the Conquest of New Spain. *His countrymen called it* la noche triste *— the night of sadness — to convey their loss and suffering. But Diaz del Castillo makes it clear where his sympathies lie: with the Aztecs, who suffered far more, because they let Cortés get away.*

The meaning of noche triste *has changed since then. It's become a metaphor for the birth of Mexico, the birth of a mestizo people — a painful birth, but a birth nonetheless. But Mexicans use the term even more broadly, to refer to any source of sorrow, to anything bittersweet. It's the defeat that lies at the heart of every victory, and the victory that lies at the heart of every defeat. It's something that appears good but is actually bad, and something that appears bad but is actually good. As you explore this enchanted land, remember this. It is a night of sadness.*

The next morning I went to the Casa Na Balom, a museum and research institute that was a well-known meeting place for people in the solidarity movement.

I joined a tour in progress, a large group of white people all dressed in sturdy hiking boots and red bandanas and army-issue backpacks, speaking to each other in

Spanish with a German accent. We followed an American woman into a gallery filled with embroidered tunics.

When the Mayan woman puts on her huipil she emerges through the neck opening into the center of the world, the American woman said.

She spread her arms to show us the design of the huipil she was wearing.

This was given to me by a woman from Tenejapa, she said. The rows of diamonds represent the movement of the sun through the heavens. The curls on each side are butterfly wings, representing the night sky. The modern Maya read these symbols just as their ancestors did. Each woman interprets the ancient patterns in her own way. This is why they continue to weave, even in the refugee camps. They're keeping this language alive. They're telling the world they will not die.

We followed her into a gallery with display cases containing skulls and burial urns and clay figurines, and into another gallery full of iron crosses. When the tour was over the Germans went to the gift shop and I approached her and asked if she knew anything about El Rosario, a refugee camp on the border, near the Lagunas de Montebello. I'd learned about it from people in the Network. They said that was where Guatemalans had fled after the massacre in San Francisco Nenton.

You have to be part of the church to work in a camp, the American woman said.

I thought they might need volunteers, I said.

She looked at me as if I were contagious.

You have no business going to El Rosario, she said.

I went to the zocalo and sat on a bench by the bandstand. My hunger pangs were coming on, the white spots flashing in my head.

When the pain had passed I opened my eyes. It was easy to see why San Cristobal was such a tourist spot, I thought, what with the white cobblestone streets, and the baroque buildings with their brightly colored facades, and the green mountains rising in the middle distance, all the way to the clouds.

I went to a couple of shops on the zocalo, looking for a bowl of miller's bran, or a tuna-fish sandwich without the mayonnaise, but there were no such things here, so I went to a café and bought a yogurt and returned to the bench by the bandstand. I ate fast, full of guilt, and right when I'd finished the Germans I'd seen at Na Balom entered the square. They walked toward me, animated, gesticulating, still speaking in Spanish. Even though I didn't speak Spanish I was certain they were talking about the camps, that they were here for the same reason I was, and were the ones I would need to talk to, the ones who would know what to do, and I hoped maybe they'd come looking for me, to tell me they wanted me to travel with them, but instead they walked right past me, and I just sat there, not saying a word.

I had come to Mexico without a plan. Not for finding food I could eat, not for finding work in a camp, not for communicating with people who didn't speak English. The American woman at the Na Balom was right: I had no business going to El Rosario. I had no business being in Mexico at all.

I went back to my hotel room and sat down on the bed and cursed myself for the yogurt. It was just sitting in my intestines now, turning to sludge, and I had no bran, no way to get it out.

I looked at the painting of the woman in the blue tunic. She was pressing her hands together, as if in prayer. She radiated a red light. Her expression was benevolent, but sad.

I assumed she had something to do with the Catholic Church, but I didn't know if she was the same as Mary, or similar to Mary, or different from Mary. I found her image comforting, which surprised me, because images of Jesus had always scared the shit out of me, even if he wasn't depicted on the cross, because I knew the agony of the cross was always there, waiting for him, waiting for me, because when I was a boy the company my father worked for transferred our family back east, to a Catholic mill town outside Boston, and the kids in the neighborhood taught me — beat it into me — that I killed Christ.

I looked in the guidebook to see if there was anything about the woman in the blue tunic and found an entry that told her story:

In Mexico the Mother of God is God and her name is Guadalupe. She appeared before the Chichimec peasant Juan Diego on December 9, 1531. He was walking from his village to Mexico City, as he did every Saturday, to attend the Sunday morning mass, dressed in his white tilma to protect him from the sun. When he reached the summit of Mount Tepeyac he heard a woman call his name and he turned and saw her standing among the prickly-pear trees. Her skin was brown, like his, and her long black hair was shining in the sun.

She spoke to him in Nahuatl, the language of his people. She said she was the Virgin of Guadalupe and asked him to go to the bishop in Mexico City and instruct him to build a church on Mount Tepeyac for her people. Juan was so stunned he couldn't speak, but he promised to do as she requested.

The next day after mass he was granted an audience with the bishop. He spoke to the bishop through a Nahuatl interpreter and explained who Guadalupe was and what she wanted. But the bishop chastised him, reminding him he had been baptized in the name of Jesus Christ Our Lord and Savior, and taken the holy communion, and that these were sacred acts. The bishop told Juan that he was committing blasphemy, worshipping a false god, because there was only one way into the kingdom of heaven, and that was through Jesus Christ. But Juan was steadfast. He insisted he had seen Guadalupe and that she had spoken to him. So the bishop asked him for evidence, some sort of proof of Guadalupe's existence, and told him to leave.

As Juan walked back to his village he felt ashamed. He was afraid to see Guadalupe, to have to confess his failure to her. As he climbed Mount Tepeyac he pulled his tilma over his head in the hopes that he might hide from her, even though he knew this was impossible because she was the Mother of God. He was so relieved when she didn't appear.

The following Saturday he set out for Mexico City, and as he approached Mount Tepeyac he again pulled his tilma over his head, but when he reached the summit she was there, waiting for him. She drew closer to him this time and touched his arm. He begged her forgiveness, and told her he had tried, but the bishop had been scornful, and questioned his conversion, and demanded proof. He told her he wasn't the right person to do this, and she said he was, that she had chosen him for a reason, that it was his belief when no one else believed that was going to convince the world. Then she said he should go to the prickly-pear trees and pick the yellow flowers and bring them to her. He did as she asked, and she arranged the flowers in his tilma, and tied it off at both ends and draped it over his neck, and he continued on to Mexico City.

The next day after mass he was granted a second audience with the bishop, who wasted no time asking him for proof of Guadalupe, and he was filled with dread, because he knew the yellow flowers would be insufficient. But as he untied his tilma hundreds of brilliant red roses spilled onto the floor, and there, emblazoned on the inside of his tilma, was the image of Guadalupe, her brown hands pressed together, her blue tunic glowing, her body encircled in a halo of red flame.

Juan's tilma, with Guadalupe's image, hangs in the Basilica on Mount Tepeyac to this day. Every year millions of people make the pilgrimage to Mexico City to see it.

Of course there are those Mexicans who don't believe the story, who talk instead about Tonantzin, an Indian god native to the region. They say the Church knew it could never convert the Indians unless it could make itself familiar to them, so it appropriated Tonantzin and renamed her Guadalupe. They say Guadalupe was a tool of oppression, an instrument for eradicating the native religion, just as other madonnas in other cultures have been. But they say they love her just the same, because the Creole clerics underestimated her, failed to appreciate her, didn't realize that in the process of remaking her she would remake them. They didn't know that she would force them to accommodate her until she reconfigured the Holy Trinity itself, until she was the God of Mexico, until she

represented a Christianity that, at the most fundamental
level, had nothing to do with Christ.

The next day I got on a bus for the Lagunas de Montebello. The road down the plateau was winding and narrow, though the bus driver was unfazed: He accelerated into every turn, until we were leaning so far over I thought we were going to roll it. He almost hit a woman who was pushing a cart stacked with corn, and a group of men with machetes who were hacking a thicket of sugarcane.

At the bottom of the mountain the driver pulled off the road and opened the door and three cops got on. They surveyed the passengers, saw I was the only foreigner, and walked down the aisle to where I was sitting. I took out my passport and a $5,000 peso note.

Not here, Flaco, they said.

I didn't know *flaco* meant thin, or skinny, or that Mexicans used it as a term of endearment, often ironically, so a wife might call her fat husband *flaco, or flaquito*. But it was clear these cops weren't calling me *flaco* to express affection.

I grabbed my bag and followed them off the bus. They led me to their car and asked me where I was from, where I was going, and why I was in Mexico.

You better not be an activist, they said.

I'm here on vacation, I said.

That's good, Flaco. You don't look like an activist.

They laughed. The bus driver honked his horn.

Show us your papers, they said.

I gave them my passport and the $5,000 peso note.

We want to see your visa, they said.

I was told I didn't need one, I said.

You were told wrong, they said.

I reminded myself this was all part of the shake-down. *La mordida*, or the little bite, my guidebook called it. It was the price of traveling in Mexico. But I was scared.

You're coming with us, they said.

The bus driver honked again. One of the cops whistled to him. He closed the door to the bus and drove away.

I took a $10,000 peso note out of my wallet and gave it to them. They laughed again.

That's all I have, I said. The rest is traveler's checks.

Comitan is just down the road, they said.

They got in their car and took off.

I reached Comitan just before dusk. Its zocalo was treeless and plain, the buildings square and white, except for the church, its terra-cotta exterior covered with stucco arabesques and sculptures of saints. There were some men on the bandstand, playing dominoes. I sat on a bench and took out my guidebook to look up hotel listings, but there were no entries for Comitan.

Oye Flaco, the men said.

I went to a little market on the zocalo and cashed a traveler's check, then searched the shelves for tuna fish. Once again I couldn't find anything, so I bought a few cans of sardines, a box of cornflakes, a lemon, and a two-liter bottle of water.

I walked the streets until I found a hotel I could afford, a place called the San Vicente. It was a cinder-block building painted green. When I checked in the desk clerk asked me how many people would be staying in the room.

Just me, I said. But my wife will be joining me in a few days.

He gave me a room key, then wagged his finger at me.

Drink water okay, he said. No toilet.

Mexico was in the middle of a long drought and people faced steep fines if they exceeded the monthly water allowance. I'd seen travel advisories about it at the airport in Mexico City and smelled the results: the shit piled up in the bus-station toilet in Tuxtla. There hadn't been any restrictions in San Cristobal — for the sake of the tourists, I now assumed.

I understand, I said.

I asked him if he had a bowl I could use and he looked at me like I had three heads. I made the shape of a bowl with my hands. He fumbled around under the counter and handed me a small foil pan.

Thank you, I said.

You eat, he said.

The room was dark and hot. There was a twin bed in the corner, with a heavy blanket folded at the foot, and a picture of Guadalupe over the headboard. There was a lamp and an old rotary phone on the nightstand. In the bathroom there was a toilet and a sink. Mosquitoes hovered over a drain in the floor.

I sat on the bed and took a swig of water. I poured some cornflakes into the pan and crushed them into crumbs with my fist. I opened a can of sardines and tore them into pieces and mashed them into the cornflakes. I took a small piece of the mixture and put it in my mouth, pressing it against my palate with my tongue to extract all the flavor, waiting until it had almost dissolved before I swallowed.

When I was finished eating I took off my clothes, lay back on the bed, and read some more of the guidebook. And then the mosquitoes descended on me.

I got up and grabbed the lamp and held it as high as I could. I saw, in the dim light, what looked like hundreds of them, huddled together where the wall met the ceiling. I stood on the bed and tried to smash them with the side of my hand, but they scattered fast. They were nothing like the mosquitoes I knew from Los Angeles, those end-of-summer mosquitoes, fat and lazy. These mosquitoes were agile and determined, and I could feel the first welts rising on my neck, and on my arms.

Fuck this, I said. I'm going to kill all of you.

I went to a corner of the room and squatted down and waited. When they were shrill in my ears I stood up, spun around, and slammed them with the guidebook, over and over, crushing some of them, bursting others, the ones that were full, the ones that had already fed on me, and felt vindicated each time my blood blotted the wall, until my welts were itching so bad that I ran back to the bed and unfolded the blanket and covered myself with it. It was made of a coarse wool that irritated my skin, but it was thick and protected me. I made a little opening for my mouth so I could breathe, and lay there, drenched from head to toe in sweat, listening to their high, frustrated keening until the early morning hours, when sunlight started to fill the room, and they relented, and went dormant, and I fell asleep.

I woke at noon and went to the bathroom. I could hear water gurgling in the drain in the floor, and it smelled like rotten eggs, and I realized there was something wrong with the septic system. Mosquitoes were probably breeding inside that pipe.

I splashed cold water on my face and my neck to soothe some of my bites, combed my hair, and got dressed.

You motherfuckers are dead, I said.

I went back to the little market on the zocalo, bought a fly swatter and a bottle of bleach, returned to my room, and poured the bleach down the drain. Then I stood on the bed and dragged the edge of the fly swatter along the line of the ceiling to scatter them, and as each one resettled on an accessible part of the wall, I swatted it. By sunset I thought I'd killed all of them, but just to be sure I squatted down in the corner again and waited for the remaining ones to come for me.

The next day I went to the Comitan bus station and boarded an old school bus for the Lagunas de Montebello. There were children sitting near the front, holding big baskets of gum with unusual flavors — menthol, eucalyptus, citron. They begged me to buy something.

Compre chicle, Señor Flaco! Por favor!

I gave them 50 pesos for a pack of tamarind.

Gracias Señor Flaco! Gracias!

Cállense, niños, the driver said.

Pajarito canta tú, canta tú, canta tú, they sang. Pajarito canta para mi!

About half an hour into the trip the driver suddenly pulled over and I felt a knot in my stomach, fearing it was the cops again, but it turned out he was just stopping for a fruit stand at the side of the road. I watched from the window as he picked over crates of mangoes and papayas. Ten minutes later he was back, his arms loaded down with green fruit that he gave to the children, and they put it in their baskets.

Pajarito conduce tú, conduce tú, conduce tú, they sang, and the driver started up the bus.

He dropped me off at the entrance to the Lagunas de Montebello, though it wasn't an entrance so much as a cockeyed sign with the words *Lagunas de Montebello* and an arrow pointing east. Sunset was still hours away, but the cicadas were already screaming.

I followed a dirt path through a field of tall yellow grass until it disappeared into a forest of pine trees. I tried to keep walking in the general direction of the sign, toward a cool breeze coming through the trees — coming off the water, I kept telling myself, even though there wasn't any water in sight — but after 15 minutes I had to admit I was lost. And then, out of nowhere, I came upon a small concrete structure with rough openings for windows and a door, and I went inside.

A woman in a red apron was sweeping the floor. I begged her pardon and asked her if she could tell me how to get to the Lagunas de Montebello. She laughed, disappeared into an inner recess, and returned a moment later with a card table. She covered it with a red checkered cloth and motioned for me to sit down.

I don't want to trouble you, I said. I just want to know how to get to the lakes.

Tell me what I can get you, she said.

You speak English, I said.

She disappeared again, and for several minutes I heard her banging pots and pans, and running what sounded like a blender, and then she came back with a bowl of black beans, a plate of nopales, a stack of fresh tortillas, and a chocolate milkshake.

Maybe it was because I didn't understand what was happening, didn't know if this was the woman's home, or her restaurant, and wanted to show my deep appreciation, and do nothing that might offend her. But as she stood there, waiting, watching, wanting me to enjoy what she had made for me, I decided to do something I hadn't done in a long long time: violate my diet.

I didn't know how much to eat, or when to stop, or what it was like to feel full, because I'd grown so used to studying my every sensation, to noting the subtlest changes in my body, so that even the slightest fluctuation, barely perceptible, felt enormous. But I scooped up the beans and the nopales with the tortillas, and drank the chocolate shake, until it was gone, all of it, and I knew, with absolute certainty, that it was the best meal I'd ever had.

You're from the United States, she said.

Los Angeles, I said.

The Dodgers are my favorite team. I love Fernando. I just wish they could beat the Reds.

Me too. I hate the Reds.

She cleared the plates. When she came back I asked her if she knew about El Rosario.

You can't go there, she said.

There were people in San Cristobal, I said. Germans. I'm pretty sure that's where they're going.

I don't know anything about Germans, she said. But it's not safe. The Guatemalan army is crossing the border at night. They just kidnapped a mother and her two daughters. They cut out their tongues and their genitals and drowned them in the Lago Internacional.

When I asked the woman how much I owed her she waved me off.

They've started taking people to a school in Palenque, she said. Before relocating them to Campeche. Maybe you could go there.

I asked her how to get back to the highway. She told me there were blue blazes on some of the trees, but they were hard to see, and spaced irregularly, so I needed to leave before it got too dark. I thanked her and gave her a hug.

You're too skinny, she said.

I didn't have sardines and cornflakes that night. I had to atone for the milkshake. I had to cleanse myself. I had to start all over again.

I got undressed, got into bed, opened the guidebook, and started reading the entry for Palenque.

Getting there is itself a magical experience. Carretera 199, like everything in Mexico, takes its own sweet time. As you wend your way across the central plateau you'll see herds of cattle and sheep grazing openly on wide green hillsides, and pass through small villages where women still wear the traditional huipils – handwoven shawls with brightly colored, intricate designs.

The ancient city will appear before you all at once, its limestone structures shining white in the oblique orange sun. From the main gate, follow the signs through a grove of magnolia trees, and within minutes you'll be standing at the foot of the Temple of the Inscriptions, the most important structure in all the Maya world. Climb its sixty-nine steep steps to the platform. This is the highest point in Palenque, and offers a spectacular view of the Sierra de Chiapas, surrounding the ruins on every side, except to the west, where the city opens onto the plain.

I was too angry at myself to sleep. I had vowed not to let food control me, and yet I had, over and over and over again. How many times had I contaminated myself? How many times had I polluted my body? It didn't matter how good something tasted in the moment; it was never worth it. Never. Food shouldn't be pleasurable. Food should be a need, not a want. People were dying — my government was killing them — and here I was stuffing my fat fucking face. I was such an asshole. I was such a fucking asshole.

I got dressed and went to the zocalo and walked around for a while to burn off the calories I'd consumed. There were strings of white lights on the bandstand, in preparation, I later learned, for *la dia de las madres*. And the men were still there, still playing dominoes.

Pinche flaco, they said.

Now the curse words in my head — those hard consonant sounds my language had given me — were directed at them: *Shut the fuck up.*

135

I went back to the hotel. I saw the light was on in the front office and went inside. The desk clerk was entering numbers in a ledger.

I just wanted to let you know my wife is arriving tomorrow, I said.

He nodded and gave me another room key.

I told her not to overpack, I said. But I know she's going to. I'm sure she'll bring one of her sailor tops. She loves sailor tops. She probably has a hundred of them. And her blue capris. And her Bay City Rollers T-shirt.

Qué qué what?

The Bay City Rollers. They were a Scottish band. She's kind of obsessed with them, to be honest. She even slept with one of the band members, I don't know which one. It was after they broke up, or reformed — I don't know what their deal is at this point — but the guy was playing at some hole in the wall in Los Angeles and she went to the show and then went home with him.

Tengo trabajo, señor.

We met in high school, you know. Someone introduced us, and I had a crush on her right away, but then she disappeared, and I didn't see again until years later. Her family moved after their house burned down, and she had to change schools. They lived in a condo next to Chatsworth Park. She felt really isolated, cut off from all her friends, so she started going for walks in the park, venturing farther and farther out, until she was crossing the county line into the Santa Susana Pass. It was spring, and she picked wildflowers, violets and poppies and Indian paintbrush. And then one day she came upon a ravine shaded by oak trees, and she took off all her clothes and lay back in the dirt and touched herself, and felt that long slow wave stretching out inside her, and then she closed her eyes and fell asleep. When she woke up it was dark, and she was scared, and she promised herself she would never do that again. But she couldn't stop, and soon the ravine was her refuge, and she went there every day after school, but not on weekends because there were too many people in the park and she didn't want to get caught. She took me there once, just to show me this place that had meant so much to her.

Por favor, señor.

We got married in Barcelona, you know. On the steps in front of *La Sagrada Familia*. Gaudi was a devout Catholic. He never finished the cathedral, but he didn't care. He just kept changing it, depending on what was going on in his life at a given moment. When you look at the cathedral it's like you're reading a man's diary.

Señor, ya, basta.

I just need to warn you: She's going to flush the toilet. Don't get me wrong: She's very committed to water conservation. She understands that water is a finite resource. We have droughts in Los Angeles too. It's not like here — they don't fine you for your total water consumption, but they'll fine you if they catch you watering your lawn, and she always says that's a good thing, because people shouldn't be watering their lawns in the first place. You live in the desert, she says. Deal with it. And I agree with her. It's just that she's more sensitive to odors than I am. I can't smell anything. Though I must tell you, every once in a while, if she has to get up early in the morning, she'll go to the bathroom and she won't flush, because she doesn't want to wake me up, and then when I get up and see her piss in the toilet it's so touching, so comforting. It's like she's left me a little love letter. I don't know if you can understand that, but it's true. I guess you can see how much I miss her. I can't wait to see her. I really can't wait. I should call her. Just to reassure her. She's worried I'm going to get to the airport late, because I'm always late for everything.

I asked him how much it cost for a long-distance phone call, making the sign for *phone* with my pinky and my thumb.

500 pesos por minuto, he said.

I've got to be on time this time, I said. I can't let her down. I don't want her standing there, holding her suitcase, thinking she made the wrong decision.

I went back to my room and called Nicole. She picked up on the second ring. I could hear the apprehension in her voice.

I want you to come to Mexico, I said. We can travel together.

I have to tell you something, she said.

I'm eating again. Just today I had a chocolate shake.

The line went silent.

It will be like it was before, I said. I promise.

I've met someone, she said.

I didn't want her to know how hurt I was. I didn't want her to feel bad, or guilty, because there was nothing for her to feel bad or guilty about. I had no claim on her — I'd effectively ended our relationship when I came to Mexico. So when she asked if she could tell me about him I said okay, because I could see how important it was to her, how she wanted to feel like she was ending things on good terms, like we were friends, and I tried to listen as best I could, but it was difficult, though I understood that he was an Englishman by way of Italy, visiting Los Angeles, and that he played the piano and looked like Peter Frampton, and I realized she must have met him while we were still together, because she was going to go back to Italy with him now, to Florence, where his father had a furnished pension they could stay in, in Fiesole, with a baby grand piano, and at night he would play for her, and she felt like her life was full of possibility, and I said I was happy for her, and that she deserved it, and that I wanted only the best for her, and then I hung up.

Tomorrow I will start over, I thought. Tomorrow I will buy more sardines and more cereal and get back on my diet. And then I will go to Palenque.

> *Feel the cool of the temple at your back, beckoning you. As you pass through the center portal, take a moment to adjust to the sudden loss of light, and wait for the images to emerge from the darkness. The story of Palenque is inscribed on these walls.*

In the first vault you will find a bas relief of Lord Pacal, Palenque's greatest leader. He holds a torch staff over his kneeling wife, Lady Apho-Hel. She's wearing a huipil woven with diamond patterns to represent the movement of the sun through the heavens, and is drawing a thorn-studded rope through her tongue, her blood staining a parchment beneath her.

The Maya priestly class engaged in these bloodletting rituals to induce visions, to reveal prophecy. But Pacal, as the divine ruler, wasn't permitted to participate in such dangerous practices. He fasted instead, sometimes for as long as forty days. In the second vault you will find a relief of one of his visions: From the mouth of a serpent rises a warrior wearing a jaguar-skin helmet. This is the earth monster, receiving and releasing the souls of the dead.

Proceed to the rear gallery. Here you will find three separate chambers. In the central one is the stairway to Pacal's crypt, ninety-one feet below the temple floor.

Long before Pacal died the Palencanos hollowed out a single massive stone to hold his body. From another stone they sculpted the giant lid. They built the crypt around the coffin, then the pyramid around the crypt, then the temple on top of the pyramid, and when he died they placed a jade *bead in his mouth, a jade bead in each hand, and a jade figurine at his feet. They covered his face with a jade mosaic mask, with eyes of inlaid pearl. They wrapped his body in a red cotton shroud and covered the inside of the coffin with red cinnabar, the color of the morning sun. Then they lowered the giant lid in place.*

The carving on the lid of the coffin is the single greatest work of art in the Mayan world: It's the figure of Pacal, at the moment of his death. He's falling into the maw of the underworld. The sacred ceiba tree grows up behind him, in the shape of a cross. Above the ceiba is a quetzal, the divine bird of the heavens.

Pacal is weightless. Everything around him is falling away. His head is pierced by the symbols of his authority: the conch shell and the stingray spine. Like the sun, he is about to be consumed, and like the sun, he will return as a god.

This imagery came to him in a dream. Fasting made his dreams vivid, but it had an even more dramatic effect on his waking life. It turned the morning glories indigo and made them smell like licorice. It gave the magnolia trees, lost against the dominant oak, so much definition that it was as if one of his royal artists had gone into the forest and adjusted the contrast on every leaf. And when he walked the halls of the palace, and ran his hands over the limestone walls, every streak of rain vibrated green to his touch, and he traced the places where the stucco had eroded, and the armature had broken away, and the original sculptures reappeared, intact.

And as he read the entry for Palenque he remembered what Nicole had told him, the long passages she'd read to him from the book about the disease, about how it heightened your sensory perceptions. He didn't believe her, but that morning, on his way to the Lagunas de Montebello, the children were holding baskets of gum and singing about birds, and it prompted him to listen to the blue and yellow finches nesting in the palm trees by the side of the highway, and for the first time he thought he could detect a pattern in their long, discursive trills.

He was sitting in the back of the bus, and the diesel exhaust smelled like carne asada, and he remembered his father — who had died when he was a boy — standing in the backyard, drunk, burning meat on a rusty grill.

His mother had always been angry, always been violent, but something changed after his father died. She'd wait for him in the hallway, and grab him by the arm, digging in her fingernails to hold him steady.

She was so proud of her fingernails. She didn't need to use fillers or strengtheners or acrylics, and looked down on women who did. He would get home from school, and find the bowls on the coffee table, filled with cigarette butts and sunflower shells, and he'd empty them, and wash them, and bring them back, and sit next to her on the couch, and they'd watch the Dinah Shore Show together. When the closing credits rolled she'd tell him to watch as Dinah waved to the camera, because if he looked closely at the backs of her nails he'd see they were fake − not real, like hers − and he'd say yes, you're right, I can see it, but really he couldn't see anything at all.

He begged her not to hit him in the face, because it was so humiliating, but she always did, as many times as she could. Then she'd dig her fingernails deep into his arm, until he made his body limp and fell on the floor and covered his head. She'd kick him in the ribs to make him get up, but he stayed down, and this made her even angrier, and she pulled his hair, but he stayed down, and she dug her fingernails into his shoulders, and dragged them down his back, and he felt the blood seeping into his shirt, and he knew the cuts would sting in the coming days, but he didn't care, because he felt safe, because he felt protected, because as long as she didn't hit him in the face it didn't matter. He could endure it. His body was just meat. His body was just flesh absorbing impact. That was all.

Maybe fasting made him feel like his body belonged to him. Maybe it gave him a way to deal with his shame, to punish himself, to release the pressure and carry on, because he didn't want to die, because he wanted to live. Maybe that's why he did it. Maybe. There was no way for him to know. The time for such insights had passed. The lack of food had distorted his thinking. If he ate more his thinking would change. If he ate more he would want to keep eating more. But he couldn't. Even if he wanted to, he couldn't. He was starving now to cope with the feelings brought on by starving. He was starving now because he had to.

Acknowledgements

I'm very grateful to the following people:

Jessica, for your counsel and support
Todd, for always being there
Lauren, for your friendship, and your perseverance
Amy, for being my reader, my editor, and the love of my life
Max, for always being my baby boy

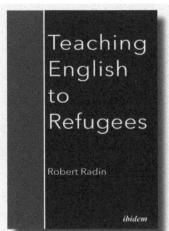

Robert Radin

TEACHING ENGLISH TO REFUGEES

03/21. 124 pages.

ISBN 978-3-8382-1502-0, Paperback   978-3-8382-7502-4, ebook
€ 22.00 [D], € 22.60 [AT], £ 20.00, $ 18.00

"Robert Radin's *Teaching English to Refugees* does it all, weaving together memoir, philosophy of language, social-justice advocacy, and graphic narrative into a haunting meditation on what can happen when the least powerful among us escape oppression and seek refuge in the United States. With the unerring precision of both linguist and poet, Radin tells a story of teaching English to refugees from such troubled areas of the world as Iraq, Somalia, and the Democratic Republic of Congo. As he struggles to find ways to reach across languages and cultures so disparate they do not even seem to be part of the same world, a quieter story plays out — his own, where multi-generational Jewish legacies get compressed into incisive and singular moments of prose you won't soon forget. Through it all, the voices of his Muslim students — haltingly at first, and then with increasing confidence — carve out a space for being all their own. Like Jenny Erpenbeck's *Go, Went, Gone*, this spare, unsparing, and intrepid book takes a close, unwavering look at some of the hardest stories of our times until nothing is what it seems at first and students become teachers to us all."

— Katharine Haake, Professor of English, California State University Northridge, author of *The Time of Quarantine* and *That Water, Those Rocks*

Robert Radin is the director of citizenship and immigration services at a prominent social-service agency in Massachusetts. His work has appeared in various publications and has been recognized in *The Best American Short Stories 2016* and *The Best American Essays 2019*.

 ibidem Press | Leuschnerstr. 40 | 30457 Hannover | Germany
Phone: +49 (0) 511 2 62 22 00 | Fax: +49 (0) 511 2 62 22 01 | sales@ibidem.eu | www.ibidem.eu

Edition Noëma
Melchiorstr. 15
D-70439 Stuttgart

info@edition-noema.de
www.edition-noema.de
www.autorenbetreuung.de